Bernardo González-Romero

The meaning of fibromyalgia

Bernardo González-Romero

The meaning of fibromyalgia

Specialized group physical therapy on a group of six persons suffering from fibromyalgia

LAP LAMBERT Academic Publishing

Publisher:
LAP LAMBERT Academic Publishing
is a trademark of
Dodo Books Indian Ocean Ltd. and OmniScriptum S.R.L publishing group

120 High Road, East Finchley, London, N2 9ED, United Kingdom
Str. Armeneasca 28/1, office 1, Chisinau MD-2012, Republic of Moldova, Europe
Managing Directors: Ieva Konstantinova, Victoria Ursu
info@omniscriptum.com

Printed at: see last page
ISBN: 978-3-659-61777-5

To Pepita

Using more words would only reduce the meaning of what I try to express as it goes beyond words.

But i hope "IT" will reach all of you.

TABLE OF CONTENTS

As professional physiotherapists we work according to our ethical codes. There are a great many political-economic and cultural actions that can prevent stress if we as PTs in our private life engage more actively.The most effective way to prevent stress is to eliminate it at its source.

Gard, G. Ph. D.

INTRODUCTION

I work in a physiotherapy unit in primary care, in public health care, in Spain. During the last years I have observed an increasing number of patients diagnosed with Fibromyalgia. As in many other places in the public health system in my country, the rheumatologists don't treat them anymore. Their services are collapsed and this illness doesn't have an effective treatment and its cause is not clearly known. Many are referred to the pain specialist unit in the hospital related with our health area, where the more powerful analgesics combined with a short standardized psychological treatment; don't prove to be efficient enough. So they come back to be treated most of the time, in our health centre by the family doctors. These patients are very time and resources consuming.With high societal cost, counting direct and indirect costs as sick leaves or early retirements.

Basic Body Awareness Therapy (BBAT) is new in my health area. It overcomes this apparent split between ``organic´´ body and mind. And it focuses on factors that support health rather than factors that cause disease. It is also new in my work setting, as far as I know. All made me think that BBAT was suitable in the case of persons suffering from Fibromyalgia in our health centre.

For one year I used Basic Body Awareness Therapy individually on persons suffering from Fibromyalgia in my center; and their Movement Quality was poor but improved and they refered more well-being.

Now I wanted to observe the phenomenon of MQ on a group setting. This is the main focus. But as a health care professional I would like to remark that this study is made in Spain, with a socio-cultural reality.The practices of medicine and psychology cannot be divorced from the cultural context in which they occur. (Van Der Kolk, Mc Farlane 1996) On the other hand much of the information used for this project comes from studies made in other socio-cultural contexts. This may ``confuse´´ the reader a bit, but I think that instead, is going to enrich this work. At the end : Today, we are all inmerse in a global culture.

This study is the final result of two years dedicated to treat fibromyalgia with this modalitie of physiotherapy in the context of primary care in public health.

After one year working with individual therapy I did a previous work with two very challenging cases (at least for me).In this work the short theory about fibromyalgia containes the basics of the mainstream scientific definition and findings. Basically: Pathofisiology but the perspective was already holistic also.I am going to add part of the work I did with this two persons after the theory chapter about Basic Body Awareness Therapy (BBAT/BBAGT) in the main content wich is about Movement quality in a group therapy work . It´s not very orthodox but I just beg the reader to focus on my observations,"surprises", the subjective and spontaneous expressions of the patients and enter with me in this "journey"which starts in this first year in contact with fibromyalgia as therapist and as person; and how the experiences and questions that I make to myself lead me to the main final research study after two years which is the main content of this book.I want to make clear that I have never been skeptical with my patients with fibromyalgia as I have shared and been aware of their absolutely real suffering. There is no intention to jocke but expressing how puzzled I felt sometimes and at the same time challenged and motivated.

At the end of the day: From the begining I always focused on the experience and result of my clinical work but I couldn´t help feeling the need to understand the phenomenon of fibromyalgia.

In the present study(once finished the "extra" of the past experience) I only focus on psychological, social, cultural and existential perspectives and findings.

The reader will find also an invitation to all of us (the health care professionals) to self-critizism that I found necessary in this topic.

Personally, I am satisfied in the sense of what I did with my patients and the improvement and result that was achieved at the end and I feel lucky for the opportunity they gave to me to lead and share all the experience with them.

Finally: Through the reading of these study it will be ``present´´ the concept of meaning. It will be not part of the research question or the main content, but the human need and search for meaning is natural and in a lived world of suffering, as is the case of fibromyalgia, is unavoidable.

BACKGROUND

The American College of Rheumatology established the diagnostic criteria for Fibromyalgia (FM) in 1990. They include: A history of widespread pain longer than 3 months and pain in 11 of 18 tender point sites on digital palpation. FM is a complex, chronic pain syndrome which causes widespread pain, aches, stiffness and fatigue as well as a variety of other symptoms .(NFP 2004). The intensity and location of the pain can vary from day to day and is also associated with sleeping disturbances. FM was recognized by the WHO in 1992. (Castellanos, S. 2012) Fibromyalgia is a chronic pain syndrome with no known etiology, cure, prognosis or clear diagnosis criteria. (Cunningham,M. 2006) No one can have fibromyalgia. Fibromyalgia is just a word we use to represent the situation of someone complaining about widespread chronic pain, fatigue, and sleep disturbance who has tender points on physical examination. It is not a disease, it's a description. (Silva 2004: 828, Journal of Rheumatology. In Barker, K. K. 2005).

Till this point we go back to "what is" and we see is hardly possible a clear agreement. And now we start to see other perspectives that will be more abundant in the theory chapter about fibromyalgia

The fact is that most of the millions of patients with FMS are women. (Barker, K. K. 2005)

A diagnosis may be significant when it provides the road to relief, understanding, or legitimization of problems. The social and medical meaning of the Fibromyalgia diagnosis appears to be more complex and seems hardly helpful after all. It does not hold the status of a medical condition which provides relief from responsibility and stigmatization. The challenge for the doctor is to tolerate the uncertainty of a diagnostic concept such a Fibromyalgia, while supporting the individual patient in using the name of the disorder to create meaning in a life of chronic illness (Undeland, M. Malterud, K. 2007).

Rosberg has studied the phenomenological meaning of the body in patients with undefined muscle tension and pain and how meaning can be created from the bodily experiences in the physiotherapy process. Multidisciplinary studies have shown that Basic BAT can increase health-related quality of life and cost-effectiveness. A group of patients received 20 sessions of BBAT and experienced a greater improvement in pain and Psychological symptoms and a more positive body image (Gard 2005). All the information in this article is about the effects of BBAT in FM and CPS. Studies so far indicate that Basic BAT has positive effects.(Gard 2005)

BBAT is a movement approach in physiotherapy. Therefore, when I decided to use Basic Body Awareness Group Therapy with persons suffering from Fibromyalgia, I decided to focus on its core concept: Movement Quality.

PURPOSE

The aim of this study is to present the promotion of MQ in a group of 6 Spanish persons suffering from Fibromyalgia, during Basic Body Awareness Group Therapy during 10 weeks. The focus will be on MQ to see what happened and how, during this period. We will focus on MQ. Analyzing the therapeutic factors in the Group Therapy, in this group, is not part of this project. But positive effects in healt-related quality of life are expected

RESEARCH QUESTION

What is the Movement Quality promotion using Basic Body Awareness therapy on a group of 6 Spanish persons suffering from Fibromyalgia, how is is this process represented and if it, as a whole, can be positive for the group?

THEORY

Basic Body Awareness Therapy

Basic Body Awareness Therapy is a physiotherapeutic method, based on the theory and practice of the French movement educator and psychotherapist Jacques Dropsy. Basic Body Awareness Therapy was developed in the beginning of the 1970's in the field of psychiatric physiotherapy by the physiotherapist, Dr. Med. Gertrud Roxendall (Skatteboe 2005). Since then, the International Teachers group has elaborated and done research for 25 years. BBAT has humanistic and holistic principles, focuses in Movement Quality and Self-exploration and Self-experience of harmonic movement. (Skjaerven, 2003) It is used clinically, for health promotion and for preventive health care. The treatment can be done with all the movements or part of them. BBAT includes lying, sitting, standing, walking, running, use of voice, interaction movements and massage. (Skjaerven 2002) The movements contain basic and universal elements that can be found in daily life. (Dropsy 1987. In Skjaerven 2002)

Norwegian P.T. modality Basic Body Awareness Therapy: focuses on the basic function of movements related to posture, coordination, free breathing and awareness that constitutes the basis for the quality of movement in action, the expression of the self, interaction with others and involvement in activities in life. The aim of BBAT is to integrate the body in the total experience of the self and to restore body awareness and body control (Gard, G. 2005)

Now we see the basics about Basic Body Awareness Group Therapy.

For Yalom, the group therapy "therapeutic factors" are effective no matter the perspective or kind of group therapy. They are eleven and are the core of group therapy. They are all interdependent and of equal importance:

1. Instillation of hope
2. Universality
3. Imparting information
4. Altruism
5. The corrective recapitulation of the primary family group
6. Development of socializing techniques
7. Imitative behaviour
8. Interpersonal learning
9. Group cohesiveness
10. Catharsis

Existential factors

This is the interpretation made by Langeland et al (2007)of Yalom´s group therapeutic factors:

1. To give hope
2. Encourage universalization
3. Share information
4. Engender altruism
5. Try new approaches
6. Develop social competence
7. Promote vicarious learning
8. Promote learning between people
9. Encourage group solidarity
10. Achieve catharsis
11. Encourage existential viewpoints.

Skatteboe was the first to establish therapeutic groups based on Basic Body Awareness Therapy in Norway. Skatteboe introduced the group therapy ``therapeutic factors´´ of Yalom (Yalom 1985) into physiotherapy and integrated them into BBAT as a basic tool in working with groups (Skjaerven 2004).Through years of practice, exploration and research Skatteboe identified the seven therapeutic factors that are most applicable to clinical work. Consisting on a set of organizing principles for groups, the therapeutic factors are: (1) Instilling and maintaining hope,(2) Universality,(3) Altruism, (4) Interpersonal learning, (5) Group cohesion, (6)

Existential factors, (7) Catharsis (not convenient or or effective therapeutic factor in Basic Body Awareness Group Therapy) (Skjaerven 2004)

BBAT is based on quantitative and qualitative based evidence.

Movement Quality and Movement Quality promotion

Based on the articles from: (Skaerven, LH et al 2008) and (Skjaerven, LH et al 2010); here is the description and figures of Movement quality and how MQ can be promoted in clinical practice.

Movement Quality in general represents a global impression of how the person moves. It covers preconditions and a range of movement characteristics. They are all interacting and interconnected processes that cannot be separated (Skjaerven et al 2008).

This total coordination embraces the four dimensions of human existence, also described as the four dimensions of quality of movement in BBAT. Each dimension is seen from a different Movement Quality Perspective.

1- Biomechanical. The spatial aspect of movement. It requires postural stability as a precondition to MQ. The characteristics of MQ that we can see are: Path and form in movement.

2- Physiological. Representing the time aspect of movement. The precondition is: Free breathing, (integrated in movement) and centering, (movement coming from the center in the trunk, which is also an inner reference). We can see: flow, elasticity and rhythm in movement.

3- Psycho-Socio-Cultural. Represents the use of energy. The precondition is awareness; to be present in the body. The characteristics of MQ that we see are: Emotional, cognitive, intentional, and socio-cultural aspects.

4- Existential. Represents personal and unifying aspects. The Precondition is self-awareness. We see the person Present in the movement, in the ``here and now´´ and MQ mirrors a sense of being whole and unified.We see also personal aspects in movement.

But MQ is also seen as a general and unifying phenomenon: Dynamic and interacting, functional, energy-saving, aesthetic, harmonic, expressing the inner state of a person and as an experience of well-being and health. This is also in the whole when we see MQ on Basic Body Awareness Therapy.

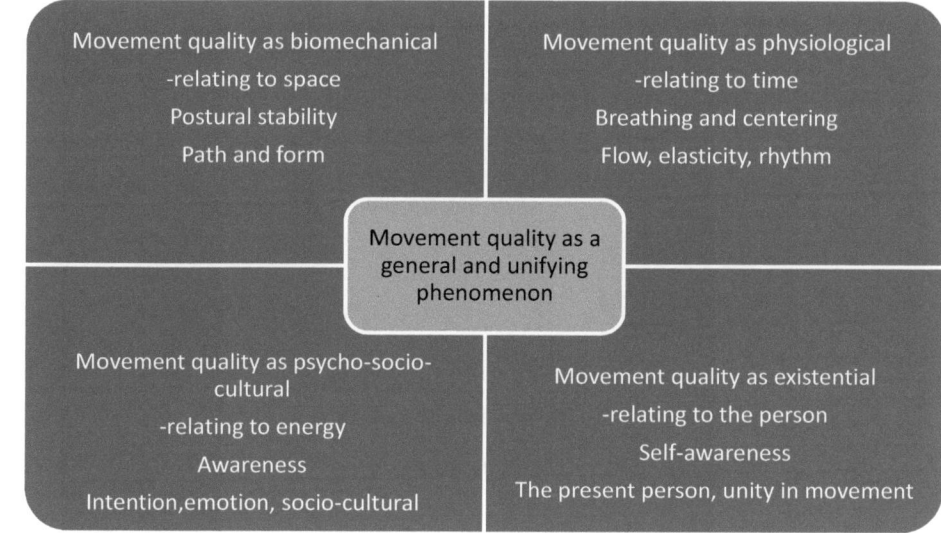

How to promote Movement Quality:

- Integrating the key elements: Balance, free breathing and awareness into the movements as a whole, we promote the general movement quality

- Preconditions for promoting Movement Quality: Embodied presence and own movement awareness of the therapist.

- A platform for promoting Movement Quality: Attitudes of trust and acceptance from the patient, building a relationship, seeing movement resources, seeing movement processes, the role of ``Father´´ and ``Mother´´ (a balance between bringing the therapy forward and try new ways and habits of moving, and listen, being calm and accepting) and creating the physical environment and atmosphere.

- Action strategies for promoting Movement Quality: Guidance versus correction, being in movement, use of words, internal and external references; and: The movement awareness learning cycle; with 7 steps: Contact (guidance to perform the movement, contact with the body), explore (in silence), experience, integrate (integrate the movement in the person), create meaning (connect the awareness training to daily life, meaning, bodily understanding), master (recognize mastering of a new and improved way of moving), reflect and conceptualize (after experiencing the movement, then find words and reflect).

The seven steps of movement awareness learning relate to each other in a cyclical form,meaning that the output of one set of processes often servs as the input for another.The therapist´s view of therapy is not linear but is a cyclical process.

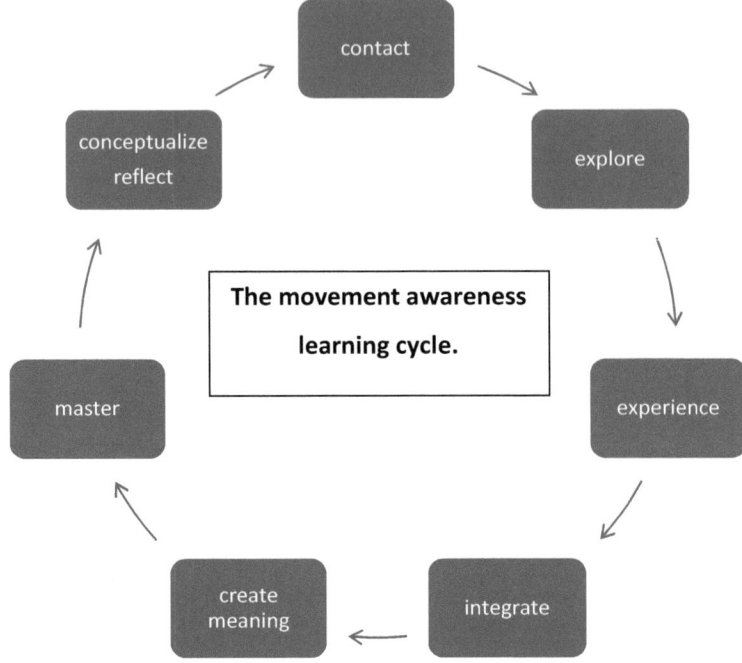

Such an approach places high demands on the physical therapist's own movement awareness. It is crucial for the therapist to become familiar with and develop movement awareness to provide appropriate guidance for patients and to pursue professional development (Skjaerven, Kristoffersen, Gard 2010).

Movement quality and sense of coherence (SOC)

Refining MQ can be understood as a process of formation of coherence in the person. In a larger existential sense, human beings search to develop a relation that opens to contact with a sense of purpose and meaningful grounds for living. A sense of coherence perceiving events in life as meaningful is health promoting. (Antonovsky 1987 in Skjaerven 2010) A person who copes well has a high SOC .(Langeland,E. 2007) SOC has ramifications at both the individual and the collective level. (Langeland, E. 2007)

Antonovsky, Salutogenesis and sense of coherence (SOC).

The theory of salutogenesis as proposed by Antonovsky(1987) represents a broader perspective on health than traditional pathogenic orientation. Antonosky does not view health as a dichotomous variable but as a health continuum, striving to explain what makes a person move towards the the healthy end of the continuum and thus increase his or Her SOC and promote coping.

The focus is on the story of thhe person rather than the diagnosis.(Langeland E. 2007)

Tension and strain are viewed as potentially health-promoting rather than illness-creating. The environment is the source of both stressors and resistance resources. The theory emphasizes the use of potential and existing resources and not only focuses on minimizing risk factors, but also emphasizes active adaptation as the ideal in treatment. (Antonovsky 1987 in Langeland E 2007)

The theory of salutogenesis distinguishes between tension and stress. When demands exceed a person´s resources or, more precisely, a person´s ability to use his or her resources, then the tension leads to stress and the person moves towards a lower level of health. Setting appropriate challenges is of great importance in creating life experiences that promote SOC and coping ability, because both overload and lack of engagement or stimulation lead to stress (Antonovsky, 1987 in Langeland E 2007).

I do think that the pathogenic orientation, which undrlines many avances in knowledge and practice, cannot explain much of the data that we have. Further, its near-total domination of our thinking has many limiting consequences. I by no means advocate the abandonment of the pathogenic orientation. My plea, rather, is that we see the two orientations as complementary and that there be a more balanced allocations of intellectual and material resources than presently exist (Antonovsky, 1987).

Sense of Coherence:

For Antonovsky, a person who copes well has a high SOC. SOC has three subdimensions.

1. Comprehensibility, or the extent to which one has a pervasive, enduring, but dynamic feeling of confidence that the stimuli deriving from one´s internal and external environments in the course of living are structured, predictable, and explicable.

2. Manageability, or the extent to which resources are available to one to meet the demands posed by these stimuli.

3. Meaning, the extent to which these demands are challenges, worthy of investment and engagement (Antonovsky, 1987). The third subdimension, meaning,

refers to the extent to which a participant feels that his or her life makes sense emotionally. Antonovsky emphasizes that this component is the most important part of the SOC concept(Langeland E 2007).

With a greater sense of meaningfulness, there is a greater sense of the other two components.The theory emphasizes four spheres in human life in wich people must invest if they don´t want to lose resources and meaning over time: Inner feelings, immediate personal relations, major activity and existential issues (Antonovsky, 1987 in Langeland E 2007)

This means that is important to be able to form a view of life (ideological, religious or political) to know people one perceives are supportive (the function of social support), to have mental stability and to be involved in rewarding everyday activities (work, sport, education etc,) (Lindstrom, 2001 in Langeland E 2007) Following (Langeland E 2007)we see other basic concept for SOC:

The general resistance resources (GRR) are crucial in the development of the SOC. GRR can be defined as any characteristic of the person, group, or environment that can facilitate tension management. The GRR are:

• Physical and biochemical: Possible link between coping with tension and immune potentiating mechanisms.

• Material: Goods such as food, clothing, and accommodation.

• Cognitive and emotional: Knowledge, intelligence, and self-identity. The theory stresses self-identity as a crucial coping resource. Knowledge gives insight and actualizes choices.

• Valuative: Attitudinal, such as coping strategies characterized by rationality, flexibility, and foresight, including active action and the effective management of emotions.

• Interpersonal-relational: People who have close ties to others resolve tension more easily than those who lack that quality in their relationships. The certainty about the availability of social support is often sufficient for this to be an effective component of GRR. Social support is a crucial coping resource.

• Macro sociocultural aspects: An individual´s culture that gives him or her a place in the world and is health-promoting and where the GRR are available at different levels (Antonovsky, 1979 in Langeland E 2007)

People who have access to and ability to utilize the GRR, in themselves or in their environment, will manage tension and perceive experiences that stimulate the development of a high SOC (Langeland E 2007).

Basic Awareness Rating Scale (BARS)

In BBAT there are three assessment tools, Motivational Analisis- Were we try to have an opinion of the patient´s motivation to avoid working against the patient´s aim. We interview in a gradual approach following 3 steps: A) Utopia- We ask him what he wants from therapy and invite him to give an answer were everything, is possible. B) Reality-We try to help by suggesting what would be possible. C) Action-Once there is a realistic plan, we focus in concrete options taken by the patient. Something like: "I am willing to do

Body Awareness Scale-Interview, wich has it´s origins in the Comprehensive Psychopatological Rating Scale from Asberg et al in 1978- It was modified by Gertrude Roxendall including some body-oriented items in 1985. It has 26 structured items.14 concern psychological symptoms, 8 concern physiological symptoms and 4 concern body attitude-related symptoms.With scores from 0(no symptoms) to 3(greatest severity)

And BARS, whose observational part is what we have used in this study.

BARS has roots in the psychiatric field and is developed by Skatteboe, Friss et al (1989)It is inspired by Functional Psychotherapy (Hart, Coriere, Karle (1989) The scale is further developed by Skatteboe (1989, 2000) and Skjaerven (1999) (Skjaerven 2002)

BARS consist of: The physiotherapist's observation of MQ in the movements, and also the patient's description of the Movement experiences after each movement.

It is developed as a tool within BBAT and consists of two parts: It is used in the observation of the harmony of the patient's movements and to promote the patients experiences and ability to communicate. (Skatteboe 2005)

BARS consist of a set of 12 movements, found to be the most discriminating between pathology and health. The choice is based on many years of clinical practice. During the 12 movements, the focus for observation is how the person is relating to the ground, the vertical axis, the movement centre, the breathing and to the expression of awareness. The movements are done in lying, sitting, standing, walking and in pair of two.

During the assessment, each movement is evaluated according to a continuous scale consisting of 7 steps, ranging from 1-7: 1 is the most pathological and disharmonic coordination, and 7 the most healthy and harmonic coordination. Point 4.0 is the midpoint of the scale; it represents the movement coordination where postural balance, the breathing and awareness meet; the unity between free flow of breathing is still weak, but possible to observe. The scale represents the four dimensions of human movement. It is possible to say that the scale ranges from the bio-mechanic perspective, the form of movement (1-3), the physiological perspective, flow, elasticity and rhythm (3-5), the psychological aspect, concerning attention, intention, emotions ending in the integration of the self/self- awareness (5-7) (Skjaerven 2002). Self- awareness is related to an existential perspective and represents personal and unifying aspects expressed in movement. (Skjaerven, Kristoffersen, Gard 2008)

The development of the assessement method is based on the central theories described by the Movement Therapist, Jaques Dropsy (1985: 1987 in Skatteboe 2005).The 3 basic co-ordinations of the trunk are an additional part of the analysis.

Based on Skjaerven 2002, BARS from 1 to 7 and the 12 movements:

1. Disharmony: The movement is stiff, staccato, dead, lack of postural stability,contact with the centre, breathing and awareness.

2. Lack of movement harmony: The movement is disconnected, mechanical and uncoordinated, insufficient postural stability and contact with the centre, breathing and awareness.

3. Weak movement harmony: The movement is a-rhythmic, still mechanical, weak postural stability, weak contact with the centre, breathing and awareness.

4. Some movement harmony: The movement has some flow, rhythm, and intention, some contact in the postural stability, some contact with the centre, breathing and awareness.

5. Moderate movement harmony: The movement has moderate flow, rhythm, expressing moderate unity and intention, moderate postural stability, moderate contact with the centre, breathing and awareness.

6. Good movement harmony: The movement has good flow, rhythm,unity, central stability and intention, good postural stability, good contact with the centre, breathing , and awareness.

7. Very good movement harmony: The movement is flowing and rhythmical, unified, free and optimally centred, very good and firm postural stability, very good contact with the centre, breathing and awareness.

The 12 movements:

1. The silent movement: The patient is lying in contact with the ground and with hands apart on contact with his abdomen (center)

2. Closing legs toghether: The patient is lying and with the legs togheter closes and open searching for contact from thighs to knees with the movement coming from the centre and following a rhythm

3. Symetrical stretching: Lying with the arms up above the head (if possible) and the patient elongates in opposite directions from hands to feet.

4. Asymmetrical stretching: The same but this time it´s only one side of the body followed by the other side. Again we search for rhythm.

5. Sitting balance: We invite to search for sitting alignment and explore gravity and stability. During this movement we invite the patient to close her lips,exhale and make the sound "MM"

6. Knee-fexing and extending:Standing we go up and down sensing the line of balance with the vertical axis of gravity

7. Sideways movement: Standing wit knees open and free the patient moves from the left to the right keeping the vertical axis and stability

8. The whipping movement: It´s a basic human movement with total coordination. Standing the patient turns around the vertical axis with the whole body including the breathing with it´´s own rhythm.

9. The wave movement of the arms: Standing we work on integrating upper and lower body around the centre of the body moving up and down while the arms forward up with flexed elbows and wrists and then low down close to the body integrated in the whole movement and rhythm; including the breathing. This movement is more complex and "looks like certain Tai-chi movemennts"

10.   Closing and opening the trunk: Standing. This movement is connected to the emotional life through it´s close connection with the breathing.When the patient goes down extends his neck and by doing it bends or closes her abdomen/centre and is invited to exhale with the sound "AAAH" going back up to the upright position.

11.   "Push-Hands": The therapist(or partner) and the patient search to realte and be sensitive to each other. They are close in a "fencer position"but with enough distance to move toghether "as only one" searching for a common rhythm forward and backwards but keeping the feet stable on it´s starting point and enough space to put in contact the outside of their wrists making a circle from centre to centre integrated in the whole movement.This is one of the relational movements.

12.   Walking: For me this is the other relational movement but from a distance. The therapist and the patient/s make a circle and start to search for this relation and sensitivity and common rhytm while focusing on the unity of the pattern of walking. We invite to lightness and free breathing.

To finish, I think it worhts for the reader to have a comprehensive overview of the historical and theoretical roots of BBAT and it´s peculiarity.

THEORY / HISTORY ROOTS SCHEME BBAT

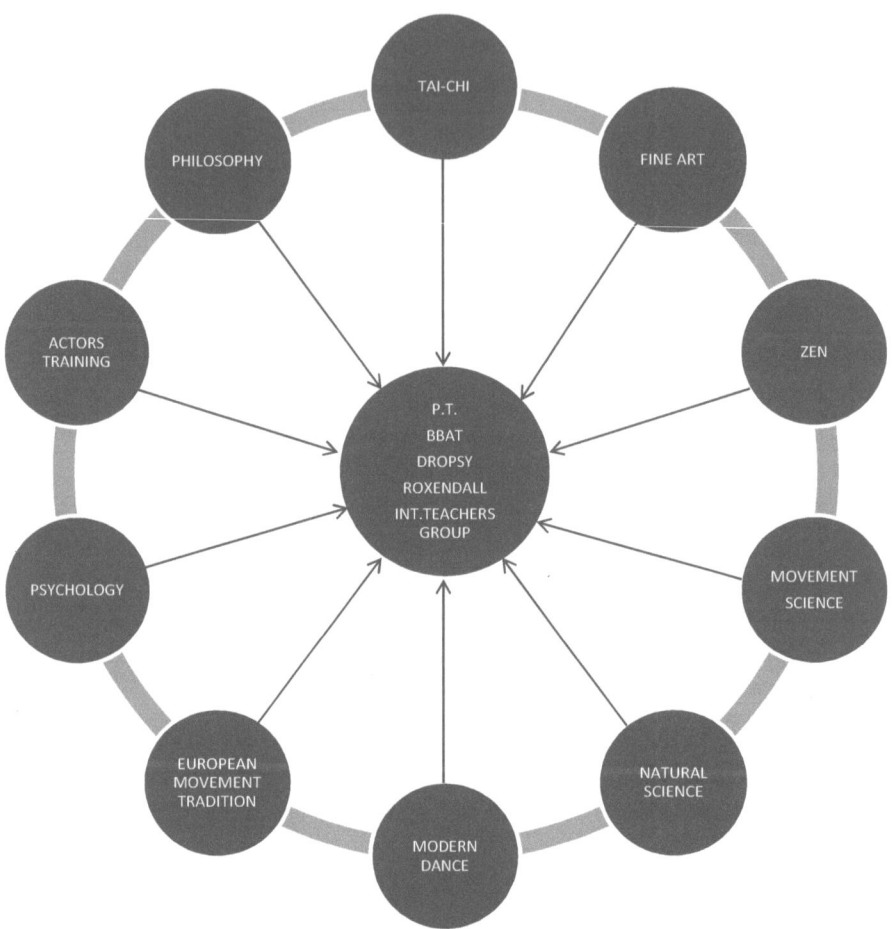

In this scheme we can see all the inspirational sources, influences and objects of study related with the history and theory of the physiotherapy's modality BBAT. We see that all these fields are of equal importance. But what I also would like to show, with the big circle connecting all of them, it's not only the fact that many of the important personalities of each field were influenced from others belonging to other fields; but the fact that many had (or have) a background in many of these disciplines. This can give us an idea of the richness and complexity of BBAT and MQ.

Fine Art as is an example: Movement teachers, dancers, and actors have studied Greek sculpture and Fine art to become aware of the richness of human movement and expression (Chekhov 1985, May, 1985 Horosko, 1991, Daly, 1996).

An important aspect of art is its function of a door opener of a tacit knowledge (Heidegger, 1996)

The case of Jaques Dropsy himself: Qualified psychoanalyst influenced by Freud and Jung, a psychotherapist influenced by Reich and Lowen. Influenced by Tai-chi and Zen; he was a mime artist, actor, dancer, choreographer and movement educator influenced by Stanislawsky, Horosko, Alexander, Feldenkrais and Bucholz.

. Between this personalities and different fields,during the last 114 years We can mention Masters like Cheng Man-Ching (Tai-chi) and Suzuki (Zen-meditation).From the western world, we have Elsa Grindler or Charlotte Selver, Feldenkrais, Alexander (European western tradition) Reich or Lowen (Psychology). Duncan and Graham (Modern dance), Stanislavsky (Actors training), Merleau-Ponty (Existential Philosophy).The use of the body to promote health, the body in psychotherapy , the psycho-physical integration, the movement and awareness for health and self – development, and the vision of the body as a whole, are concepts that are present in health and society today.

And finally: I find important to point that many of these personalities had a personal experience of suffering and quite possibly,this deep self- experience gave them a broader understanding of human existence.

"A break" to remember Ramón and Ramona

This was the short theory about fibromyalgia for me a year before the current moment after one year of individual therapy ending with the two more challenging cases that the family doctors suggested to me: Ramón and Ramona

THE FOUR DIMENSIONS OF HUMAN EXISTENCE WITH FM/FMS. THE SEARCH HAD STARTED.

-PHYSICAL: Muscle tension/spasm, weakness, fatigue, widespread pain, somatic complains, tender body areas, stiff joints. (D.A. Marcus, A. Deodhar 2011)

-PHYSIOLOGICAL: Sleeping disturbances, autonomic dysfunction, gastrointestinal symptoms, senso-neurological disturbances, changes in hormones and neurotransmitters, changes in neural structure and function, central sensitization. (D. A. Marcus, A. Deodhar 2011)

-PSYCHO-SOCIO-CULTURAL: Increased of the prevalence of FM in persons with a lower level of education and lower social class. Another data of indirect economic repercussion is the low rate of active work among FM subjects, with many people on sick leave and the large amount of women dedicated to home tasks.(A. J Mas et al. 2008) Loneliness scores were highest in patients with FM. Younger age, lower education and not working were associated with more loneliness .(M B. Kool. R. Geenen 2011) Distress, anxiety, depression. (D. A. Marcus, A. Deodhar 2011)

-EXISTENTIAL: Low responsibility, low personal energy, little joy of life and limited insight into self and existence are some of the features of the "new diseases" that make them difficult to cure, also when it comes to holistic medicine. (Ventegodt, S.Gringols, M. Merrick, J. 2005) Pain hits in the first place in the continuity of existence (Vrancken 1989) Unhomelikeness is a mode of being-in-the-world following illness, where the experienced changes in the lived body means changes in the meaning structure of one´s existence (Svenaeus 2000)

The collection of data was taken from: BARS, BAS-I, MA, reflections of the patients, observation including their spontaneous reactions, and notes after each session.

RAMON: Is a male (53) diagnosed with FM by a rheumatologist.Reired. He is also being treated by his family doctor for obsessive-compulsive disorder, intrinsic asthma, osteoarthritis, osteoporosis and psoriatic arthritis. We have made a contract with two sessions per week during the following dates: May- 3, 7, 10, 14, 17, 21, 24, 28, 31. June-4, 7, 11, 14, 18, 21, 25, 28. July-2, 5, 9, 12, 16, 19, 23, 26, 30. He had 4 sessions before making the contract as when he came for the first time he couldn't even lie, sit, or stand without pain. During this time i have made myself sure that he was ready for BBAT. I transmitted him the idea of collaborate with me but feeling free. To be in the "comfortable, well-being, pain-free zone" without "wright or wrong" and no goals or efforts but feeling well and explore on his body; either during the BBAT movements or the spontaneous movements. "Listen" to his body and stop or take "any" comfortable position even before pain happened, just if feeling the pain was coming up. This approach during 4 sessions made a moderate but immediate positive change. As he had a good feeling after the sessions and he really wanted to come back and I decided I could keep him safe; we made the contract. From the beginning I encouraged him to practice the movements during his normal life but I didn´t push much as he always answered with a lot of problems and difficulties to do it. Still: I insisted during the sessions (just reminding and suggesting it as something that would reinforce our work and be useful in daily life).On his FIRST MA the results were : Utopia-"Fix the world". Reality: " Get rid of pain and be more useful for my family". Action: "Do BBAT seriously." On his first BAS-I he scored in the more pathological level in all items and reported taking an uncountable number of drugs. On his first BARS I saw a Disharmonic Movement Quality, with peculiarities in some movements, this and his own descriptions were the base to organize the pattern for the future set of treatment sessions. In the silent movement:Big compensation in neck (needed a very big pillow) and also smaller compensations in knees and shoulders. There was no rhythm on his breathing but he yawned constantly with a big movement from the centre and he had certain awareness: ("I forget about everything around me, I feel calmed, disconnected and I breathe better").In the sitting balance he couldn´t stay on the axis and there was no unity while searching and also reported pain but surprisingly, he was feeling pretty well during the "M" sound, with a moderate pitch and volume and an increased awareness. Still: he had to support his back in a chair and he closed his eyes. About standing up and down… we didn´t even try it (only by mentioning it and seeing me, he was feeling pain and tiredness). With the sideways movement there was no flow, rhythm, no contact with the axis, stiffness with no dissociation upper/lower body, his arms were rigid in a mechanical movement and I couldn´t see free or integrated breathing. But he enjoyed it. With the whipping movement he had a certain stability related to the axis, but the movement was not coming from the centre (only upper body) On the periphery, his arms were rigid. But his description was: "I feel pain but I also feel that I can diminish it. I find it interesting. I want to search". With the wave movement of the arms there was a low stability related to the axis; no integration movement/breathing or upper/lower body. Almost no flow, rhythm or awareness (no concentrated or present). He overanalyzed the mechanics of the movement calling it "tired and uncomfortable", but "psychologically: relaxing and making him feel peace and quietness…like flying". With closenig and opening the trunk he had no stability related to the axis, moderate integration upper/lower body and too much energy in the movement. I only did it because finally he understood that we had to be present with all our body, feeling and exploring with all our body´s senses. I was afraid of a fall due to his tendency to close his eyes and lean backwards. On the other hand he was feeling "breathing really free" and "releasing tension". The "A" sound was present (short time and low volume). There was a big compensation opening his knees. There was no pain and, as he gained stability; i decided it was safe. With "push hands":Just trying was too much psychological pressure for him, causing stress and pain. Also discarded. During walking in circle there was no coordination and his head was leaning a bit forward (out of the axis) but he had rhythm and presence ("I feel like forgetting my pains and leaving all behind. I really enjoy it")

The following sessions were organized as follow: Starting point (sitting with "M" sound, his second favorite) then the sideways movement,whipping movement,closing and opening the trunk (with intervals back to initial position to avoid tiredness and pain on the patient); then sitting with "M" sound increasing his feeling of well-being and ending on with the silent movement(his favorite). He had a very laborious and painfull process to lie down and stand up in this last part of the session that improved with my advice that he had to "listen to his body" to do it avoiding pain, breathing free and with no hurry) At the end of the whole session he was feeling very well. As experienced P.T. I had so many times the temptation to tell him the" easier and best" way to do it!!. As he was doing "contradictory" movements, naturally , even enjoying them, without pain; but "unthinkable"; because they were far ahead of his supposedly knees flexion pain- free range of movement and limit during the sessions. As far as we were on BBAT, i didn´t do it because I thought that following this process will be better in terms of finding self-efficacy by himself, being a benefit for all aspects of his life. During the sessions till the next BARS (7-july) There is a certain improvement in his MQ .There is a freer and a bit more integrated breathing with glimpses of rhythm on it sometimes; and an increased awareness (more concentrated in the movements and less need of verbal communication during movement).We were making small improvements day by day but the patient made also interesting descriptions and took decisions along with surprising reactions: "I feel my hair stand on end sometimes just when I enter the room". "I feel like bugs or electricity in my scalp (while he was scratching himself and always after the silent movement and walking in circle). "I like it and when I come with a headache it disappears". "I want to confess you something that for me is very important: I am feeling trust with you and this helps me a lot". "I don´t feel my face, it is numb, and I like it. I don´t feel tension; even in my jaws" (silent movement) "Going to the shopping center, almost forced, by my family used to be a torture but now when I sit in the car I close my eyes and start the "M" sound; I sit outside the shops and do my "M" sound and I am OK. I could even stay longer.I even forget about my family!!" Sometimes my wife and son have to call me because I don´t even know that they are there, and the same happens to me at home with silent movement". One day he brought and started to use a pretty smaller and thinner pillow than the one he used before. Another day when we finished instead of standing up and talking with me before to go, he started and holded a conversation with me very relaxed….. in full squat position!!. He always used a chair to lye back (because of his back he said) and I used the stool, leaving another one close to the wall. One day he asked me: "Why do you use a stool"?. I said: " it´s just the way they do it up there in Norway, feel free to use whatever you want". He took the stool, sat and he was immediately stable in the vertical axis with no problem and we continued with the session. The last BAS-I , MA and BARS were done the 1 and 4 of July. On LAST BARS, the patient shows a Mostly dysfunctional MQ with some functional MQ in some of the movements performed during the sessions. We try the up and down standing and it´s impossible again. But when he is doing the flexion and extension of the trunk standing, he has an almost a lack of movement harmony but he is not aware that he is actually doing the up and down with nearly a moderate movement harmony. There are some interesting descriptions: "Now I have learned what I can do and I also feel my breathing like having bigger lungs""There is no pain". He is present in the moment and living the movement; and he surprises me this day with a very powerful, long "A" sound (almost like a big shout) He says after, that he has felt "rebellion, release and forget about everything" "I feel freedom" . And at the end of this BARS he made an interesting description: "in my bad moments now I have BBAT as an alternative". The last BAS-I showed changes. Psychological: 1, 2, 3, 3, 2, 1, 2, 3, 2, 3, 3, 2, 2. Physiological: 2, 2, 2, 2, 0, 1, 3, 1, 3. Body attitude: 3, 2, 3, 0. The last M.A: Utopia: "Avoid the suffering of my family and avoid the World War III". Reality: "not to be so sensitive and have less mood changes and emotional lability". Action: "Keep coming to unload weight, and not to cry here"

RAMONA: Is a female (48) diagnosed with FM by a rheumatologist. Unemployed. She is also being treated by her family doctor for depression, migraine without aura, varicose veins, repeated episodes of sciatica and cervical brachial syndrome. Her family doctor remarks that she is in the process of divorce (her husband left her for another woman) , but for "economic reasons" they lived in the same household for almost a year. It caused a traumatic relationship with psychological hostility and abuse by her ex-husband. Her daughter (17) also suffered the impact of this relationship and ended up suffering a depression. Her family doctor says that since all this happened, all the symptoms related with her fibromyalgia aggravated. She starts to have social support as her family now accepts that she has a health problem. On the other hand: She is living with her daughter who doesn´t accept it and has a "selfish behavior"(reported by the patient). We have made a contract with two sessions per week during the following dates: May- 2, 7, 9, 14, 16,

21, 23, 28, 30. June- 4, 6, 11, 13, 18, 20, 25, 27. July- 2, 4, 9, 11, 16, 18, 23, 25, 30. She had 4 sessions before making the contract as when she came for the first time she couldn't even lie, sit, or stand without pain. During this time, I made myself sure that she was ready for BBAT. I transmitted her the idea of collaborating with me with the knowledge that she already had of her body; to be in the "comfortable, well-being, pain-free zone" without "wright or wrong" and no goals or efforts but feeling well and explore. It made an immediate positive change and in the second session all the major problems seem disappeared and she wasnted to do all the 12 movements except the sideways. As she had a good feeling after the sessions, she really wanted to come back and I could keep her safe; I decided to make the contract. I encouraged her from the first session to practice at home but, as far as she always told me that it was too complicated in his normal life, I didn´t push much (but suggested it very often during the treatment. As something helpful).She improved at the end of the sessions, but Ramona´s breathing had very little freedom from the beginning, with a very small movement in the centre and with no rhythm (long periods without movement on it during the silent movement). Finally she got some rhythm. It has been one of my biggest problems when I have tried to evaluate her MQ progress. Only in the last two sessions, she started to sigh during the silent movement. If I look at the scores and the movements variables, she would have some (or even moderate) MQ and she reached this level in not too many sessions, but I haven´t been able to "see" her breathing and have an impression of how free and integrated it was on the movement (only a few glimpses during the "M" sound and the "A sound"). My only clear reference was during the pair movement: Here, her breathing was deep, clear, audible and with a rhythm almost like mine. Many positive descriptions from the patient will be seen now with the two BARS, BAS-I and also some descriptions and reactions from Ramona that have been perplexing, difficult to interpret and very challenging for me.

Ramona has been very enthusiastic from the beginning. During the closing-opening of the trunk invited to the "AAH" sound she was feeling something inside her centre that she rejected and couldn´t expulse. Finally she said that she was feeling frustrated because it didn´t happen and she didn´t wanted to do this movement although she always liked it. I stopped it and encouraged her to do it on her own and try again with me whenever she wanted. One day she came as usual and after the movements lying on the ground,when I invited her to stand, she stopped and said very determined:" I don´t want to stand up and I don´t want to go , and I don´t want to follow the session. I have lost my faith". I felt like receiving a chess-mate!. I am not trained for verbal therapy and this is not my goal, I invited her to breathe and go back to the silent movement. She did it but she talked for half an hour(I just listened and basically she was talking about her life, her problems) then stood up, told me that "she had found a source of energy with BBAT", and left.It only happened once but I felt very challenged and worried about the course of the treatment as far as she hardly ever neede the "role of father" from me. One day she came and dived headfirst into the mat (and i mean it) shouting: "This is my time"(with no pain at all!!). At the end of this session and after our spontaneous stretches she told me with a big smile: " I can do more things that you can imagine". How could I doubt it?. I wouln´t have landed on the mat like her without previous training!. She had a meeting with her sisters for them to give her support and started to change things in her apartment. She came to the last BARS session on a Saturday. As she arrived she said with a temper: "All what I need is money and I could be perfectly!!"; then we started and everything was going well, suddenly, when we were about to finish the last 3 movements;suddenly and with no previos expression of pain or tiredness, she sat on the floor, started to scratch intensely all her legs and said that they couldn´t work anymore cause they were, tired and in pain. I just asked her for her descriptions thinking in the last session when she experienced the last 3 to "complete the subjective part of BARS along adding my latest observation of her movements" But in fact, her MQ had decreased a lot..Then, she stood up for a while, and asked me to do the pair movement (even in pain, she said, " because of the energy") and when we finished, she left walking as fast as an athlete. I have to add that in this last session she asked me if she could do the "M" sound in all the movements when practicing at home, and I had to ponder very much; answering her that: "yes, you can (I thought that by doing it somehow she was integrating breathing with movement and exploring) but you also should practice the same way we were doing on therapy". And when we were going to do the sideways movement, on the second BARS, (that was discarded after the first BARS, as far as she couldn´t even try, not even two seconds, because of the immediate pain and tiredness); she told me openly that she had been practicing it regularly on the train (from the very beginning).

FIRST MA. Utopia: "Be able to change my life. Going to the middle of nowhere and have a house/farm and be self-sufficient" Reality: " Get a job" Action: "To came here to reduce my pain and gain power and help me to think". SECOND MA. Utopia: "Less pain, more energy, get a job, less limitations. Study Social integration and help (the immigrants as an example)". Reality: " having less problems, having a salary for me and another for my daughter for her to keep studying, travel and see the world".

Action: "Keep doing what I can". On the FIRST BAS-I, every single answer is accompanied with all pathological descriptions related with pain, with her organic body described " piece by piece". Psychological: 2, 3,0, 1, 0, 1, 3, 3, 3, 0, 0, 0, 3, 2. Physiological: 1´3, 1, 1, 2, 1, 3, 0. Body attitude: 3, 1, 3, 0. On the SECOND BAS-I; she jokes openly for the first time; during, and at the end of it. Psychological: 1, 3, 0, 1, 0, 1, 0, 3, 3, 0, 1, 0, 1, 2. Physiological: 1, 2, 0, 0, 2, 1, 0, 0. Body attitude: 0, 2, 0, 0.

FIRST BARS. N-1-Disfunctional movement quality.There are no compensations (she uses a soft mat for babies of less than 1 cm of thickness which ends up being a few millimeters under her head).Almost no freedom on her breathing with little movement on the centre, without rhythm (long moments without movement). And little mental awareness. " I feel well but my mind comes and goes with a lot of things that I have to organize".In the symmetrical stretching"I feel mentally unbalanced and shaky but I feel tickling and kind of massage on my female organs". In the asymmetrical stretching "I feel like if I were split in two; like if I were separated in half, from the centre. It´s pleasant, and if I can do that with my body, maybe I could do with the rest of it "(she talks about arms, legs, neck etc.). In the sitting balance the vertical axis is unstable, the movement has no unity and is mechanical, there breathing has very little freedom and the "M" sound is present in only two attempts that end up frustrating her being all the time almost no awareness. Still she wants to keep doing the movement in the future as she is sure that even though she has no "capacity"; she likes the inner vibration. In the wave, no vertical axis axis, no integration upper/lower body or movement/breathing, relative rhythm, flow and certain awareness. "I feel relief, it fills me". Closing-opening the trunk: No postural stability relative to the axis, poor integration upper/lower body and movement/breathing. No "A" sound and little awareness. " I like it; but I feel something strange in my abdomen, like if I wanted to get something out or I had something inside and I couldn´t do it". In the "push hands"The circle is very small, I feel her arm like "defensive". The stability and balance relative to the axis is not good. The movement is not centred. There is a relative integration in the whole movement. "I am not afraid of the movements; it´s just I don´t accept myself as a person. I don´t accept the way I am" " I like this movement, my body responds more to pair it with another. I feel relaxed and I don´t feel pain " About walking(with very poor MQ)" I like it. I feel comfortable"

THE LAST BARS. Silent movement: Her breathing is slightly freer, more movement, stops for short periods but there is a more regular rhythm and, for the first time, she stars to sigh . More awareness (her body is completely quiet and forgetts about her glasses, also for the first time). " I feel freedom, my mind empty and my face relaxed". In the rest of the movements on lying position remains the same as before but she can hold and increase a bit the rhythm and tempo. " It´s easier for me. I feel relief. Is like if my body was elongated/stretched like if I were in one of this medieval torture devices".There is an "M" sound with low pitch, small volume and very short time. There is certain awareness (" I escape from everything"). On standing:" I like it. I feel some kind of benefit and I don´t feel pain". The whipping movement: Good postural stability related with the axis, the movement is initiated from the centre. The breathing is hardly visible or audible but there is flow, rhythm and awareness (unity and fully involved in time and space). " I feel good and I feel my legs more"). In the wave: "I feel pain but I like it". Opening-closing the trunk: No coordination around the centre, bad postural stability. There is a relationship between the movement/breathing and the "A" sound (short and with low volume), little flow and rhythm and little awareness. " I don´t like it anymore. I can´t express myself, there is something inside that doesn´t go out; i just can´t". But as she seemed not to want to accept this frustration she said: "I have to do it more! "I just told her that she didn´t have to do it; only when she were feeling like that. With or without me. In push hands: Little stability, certain integration in the centre, integration of the whole moving person, more opened hands circle with a more gentle sensation. Her breathing is free, deep, audible, with rhythm and integrated with the movement. "I like it. I feel like if you were giving me energy". Walking-Good postural balance and stability, I can hear her breathing. There is a certain coordination in the centre. It takes time but finally she has awareness and presence and her movement becomes easier and finally we meet on the common tempo. "I just let myself go, I feel my arms loose, the steps. I do it very often and it helps; relaxes my arms and legs and I feel very well. It´s my favorite".

Result.

. I have felt satisfied as I think my patients have improved. I think that the treatment of FM/FMS must be a long term treatment (at least on these two cases). I think that after this individual treatment, group therapy could add possibilities for improvement (whenever the patients were ready and keen on it if this ever happened at all). I have tryed to give time to my patients, adding small successes to the process .Trust is very important for the patient. You have to be adaptable from the beginning, besides any minimal change in these two patient´s life outside the room, has proved that can affect the evolution of the treatment from one session, and sometimes I could say, to the whole plan. My patients have been "unpredictable" sometimes. On occasions this is very rewarding, but sometimes I have felt like "a young priest about to lose his faith" on his mission in Spain

Discussion.

. Based on the information and the experience I have now; I just suggest: Fibromyalgia is "quite a well-defined scientific diagnosis" of a disease (without medical evidence), which is practical, permits manuals, and standardized procedures and requires from the health-care professional, the knowledge of the latest EBM research in FM pathophysiology and EBP (in a hierarchical position).. But the fact, is that this increases the gap between the clinical practice and the individuality of the human being as a whole; the living body in pain. Subjectivity, clinical judgment and stories become marginalized. (Martinsen, k.).One of the most interesting findings of the study is precisely, having found persons who fulfill completely the criteria for FM who live their lives without seeking medical help. (A. J. Mas et al 2008). I just wonder: What if nobody told the patients they had FM ?. What if they never even had heard about this word ? The treatment/therapy starts with the very first words on the first encounter. Telling,unilaterally: "You have an illness with many symptoms, whose cause is unknown, unpredictable evolution and it has no cure"; doesn´t help much. Maybe, a bidirectional holistic conversation; could promote a better prognosis. After such a beginning, then you give the best treatment, but from the best starting point. Still, in many of the multi-disciplinary programs there is a part: Education. What kind of education? Giving the patient bio-medical information, increasing the burden of the diagnosis, and adding external palliative resources ? Or maybe focusing on inner resources?

Conclusion.

Every patient has his own FM disorder. Group work must be an enormous challenge. Could it be our western society FMS disorder promoting ? In our health care systems it should be a sign of alarm.

Now after this retrospective vision, we go back to the current work after one more year, this time with group therapy, focused, more mature, with a clear research question and well defined perspectives to try to understand the phenomenon of fibroyalgia. We continue with the theory about fibromyalgia as I "see" it now.

Theory about fibromyalgia: A psychological, social, cultural and existential perspective. Searching for the meaning of "fibromyalgia" or fibromyalgia as a "search for meaning"?

In recent years, a number of "new diseases" has emerged. These are suspected of being lifestyle diseases that are particularly characteristic of our western culture. The best known are whiplash, fibromyalgia and chronic fatigue syndrome. These diseases appear to be nonexistent in many indigenous cultures, such as those in Africa, and the cause of these diseases is a mystery. The "new diseases" are characteristically vague, which makes them technically difficult to diagnose. In addition, they seem to be related to some intense, peculiar and inscrutable personality disorders that can make the patient look like one major apology for existing or even a social outcast who is just looking for a good alibi to avoid all social and human commitments. Accordingly, many physicians do not recognize the "new diseases" as being real diseases and understand them as mere social problems or personality disorders.(Ventegodt. 2005)

A comparison of the FM groups with high and low scores showed that those with low SOC scores perceived less well-being than those with high SOC scores. The FM women with a weaker SOC rated themselves significantly less hopeful. (Soderberg, S. et al 1997) Here we can remember now the importance of Meanig and GRR for the SOC concept.

Individuals with FM who have experienced traumatic life events may be predisposed to greater pain-related restrictions than those who have not experienced trauma. (Przekop, P. et al 2010) Trauma may have lasting effects on stress and health in women with FM .(Smith, B. W. et al 2009)

The prevalence of PTSD among the FM patients in this study was significantly higher than in the general population. Women with FM and PTSD reported a greater number of past traumatic events than their male counterparts. This study shows a significant overlap between FM and PTSD, according to the currently accepted diagnostic criteria for each.(Cohen, H. et al 2002)

FM has been associated with various traumatic events (Amir et al, 1997), including physical trauma and sexual abuse .(Walker et al, 1977 in Zavestoski et al 2004)

The aftermath of CSA affects the whole person, and many of the``victims´´ or``survivors´´presumably are living with some kind of post-traumatic stress disorder. (Van Der Kolk 1994 in Mattsson, M et al 1998) Trauma can affect victims on every level of functioning: biological, psychological and spiritual. (Van Der Kolk, Mc Farlane 1996)

I suggest the reader to associate trauma with the more vulnerable part of the population.

Now we are going to see part of the theories of the family doctor and Lacanian psychoanalist Santiago Castellanos.

The Isabel de R. case presented by Freud in 1895, could be considered as a XIX century FM's case.This suffering is not new, what is new is its enormous increase. FM is not an homogeneus entity. What medicine names as FM, the psychoanalysis has to considerate as a complex suffering; a transclinical condition.

The systems of assessment, quality and produccion established for industry are decanted without mediation to the attention of patients. The result is pathetic. It not only cause enormous problems in the attention of patients but it´s also the origin of deep stress between medical professionals. In this scenario it doesn´t only disappear the subjectivity of the patient but also the subjectivity of the medical doctor himself.

The exclusion of subjectivity has its consecuences. These women found themselves in an hostil health care system that can´t respond with an effective treatment. There is also a deep stress beacause they don´t feel welcome and understood, because the doctor, in his function, very often ends backwards when it comes to listening the suffering words of the patient.

The subjectivity of the patient is foreclosed and the only thing that can be expected is that the same discourse of science found a solution. The patient is just a viewer of the avatars of scientific research and there is no subjective implication.

It´s a comfortable position but full of stressing experiences. The wait is too long because from start, the discourse of science is operating with an incapacity which is proportional to the arrogance in which it manifests.

In the clinical treatment of FM is fundamental a work of articulation and collaboration between psychoanalisis and medicine. It´s about avoiding fast solutions and avoid iatrogenic.

In the clinical treatment of FM we will find the problem of stigmatization of diagnosis, with patients that after a long journey through the health system end up identyfing themselves with the system itself,downloading their own subjective responsibility.

It´s fundamental to differentiate if the somatic symptoms belong to neurosis or psychosis (Castellanos, S 2012). When Castellanos uses the word"psychosis" he refers to what is called in Lacanian psychoanalisis as "ordinary psychosis", a psychosis without exacerbated symptoms that may need hospitalization and permits a "normal" relationship with the environment. Still this diagnosis is very serious as it is any other in FM for Castellanos, that warns us that FM can in some cases, eventually, be related with suicide.

The cognitive-behavioral therapies, that try to stablish their hegemony, are fundamentally oriented to pain adaptation, placing patients in a dead end. If medicine has no adequated treatment, then the psychologist what has to do is a treatment for the patient to live with pain, without asking about it´s function and the possible relationship whith his or her life´s events.

It starts with a standardized treatment similar to all patients while on the contrary, psychoanalisis works on the singularity.

On the other hand, the subconscious is not an object that can be operated from a scientifical or technical perspective, this information not only scapes to the discourse of sience, but also to the subject himself/herself.

The techniques and advices established by the CBT are not usefull as they not consider the pshychic coordenates where the chronic pain is originated and stablished.The symptom has to be mobilized according to the logic of psychoanalisis.

It is possible a solution distinct to the adaptation to pain (Castellanos, S 2012).

Now after this perspective from a family doctor and psychoanalist with 13 years on research about fibromyalgia in primary care in Spain, we continue with psychological, social and existential research findings.

Several psychosocial factors, such as belonging to a lower socio-economic group, being an immigrant, living in a compromised housing area,having a lower educational level, experiencing lower social support and having a family history of chronic pain, were associated with the populations with FM. (Bergman,B. 2005)

Differentation of the self is a product of emotional processes within one's family of origin. One´s level of differentiation is one´s degree of adaptability to stress. The participants' levels of symptom severity could be predicted by their level of differentiation and appraisal of stressful life events occurring within a year prior to the age of onset. The level of perceived stress was the predictor variable that accounted for the greater amount of variance associated with FMS symptoms (Murray Jr.T.L. et al 2007).

It is likely that the degree to which psychological stress affects pain and, conversely, pain affects psychological stress is largely mediated by personal factors such as cognitive and affective style, behaviors and habits, social support, cultural context and other uniquely individual characteristics. (Hasset.A. L, Clauw, D.J. 2011)

The erosion of the self and life world is even more pronounced for those suffering from illnesses that lack biomedical-and thus cultural-legitimacy. Biomedicine has paid insufficient attention to issues of gender when it comes to FMS. (Barker,K.K. 2005)

The consecuences of severe social restriction on self-identity are profound. Instead of the complex and elaborate social world in which the self becomes constituted via social actions, interactions, and performance, the world of those who suffer from FMS atrophies. (Baker,K.K. 2005)

Living with FM means an existential breakdown in the familiar world first and foremost related to the lived body, with loss of bodily based integrity, control, and freedom to act. (Raheim,M. Haland,w. 2006)

Consciousness of self is an integral part of being human. Illnes self-concept (ISC) is the extent to which individuals are consumed by their illness. FM patients are more vulnerable to negative ISC. In the case of FM researchers have noted that both early developmental factors and traumas may be implicated in the onset and course of FM. Imbierowicz and Egle (2003) have found a higher prevalence of childhood adversity in FM. These adversities may help to explain why for some individuals an ordeal or illness becomes central to the self (Morea, J. M. et al 2008).

Summing up Theory

Basic Body Awareness Therapy has been presented. Related with the research question: The phenomenon of Movement Quality and how it is promoted has been described, along with Movement Quality's relationship with sense of coherence and the theory of salutogenesis from Antonovsky. Basic Awareness Rating Scale; the assessment tool used to evaluate MQ in this study has also been defined with a personal overview of the twelve movements, along with the assessment tools BAS-I and MA.We have seen also an overview of hystorical and theoretical roots of BBAT."Breaking" the structure of this work we have seen a gap between the theory related to BBAT and BBAGT and the theory about fibromyalgia containing a retrospective part from a year before with the experiences, observations and descriptions from the relationship of a physical therapist with two patients in individual therapy that has made possible the whole book. Immediately, follows as we said, the more updated chapter on theory about fibromyalgia closing the theory chapter of and focusing more on psychological, social, cultural and existential aspects and research findings; than just the physical or physiological.

METHOD AND MATERIAL

METHOD

This is a combined quantitative and qualitative study. Qualitative research can enhance both the accuracy and relevance of quantitative research. (Black 1994 in Hammel K.W. 2004)

The quantitative method emphasizes on objectivity, uses standardized methods and predeterminated designs and procedures. The aim is being able to generalize from sample to larger population. Quantification and statistics are very related with reliability (Van Den Bergh 2011).

The phenomenological qualitative method, has been used. Qualitative methods are used to obtain knowledge about the characteristics, complexities and interrelationships of phenomena, often specific human matters such as experiences, emotions, beliefs and motives (Malterud, K. 1993).

The number of participants is small, there is only one group, and the period of therapy was small. Aiming to give a broader perspective, and a more consistent answer to the research question the quantitative method that has been used, complements the phenomenological approach of the qualitative method followed in this study

Movement quality promotion in basic body awareness group therapy is something very challenging and to get a more comprehensive understanding of the whole in the result; Instead of taking the patient's descriptions during BARS or during the sessions, as data for this study; open questions including those inviting the patient to reflect about the whole process, have been chosen.

Quantitative assessment of MQ:

BARS has been used to observe and assess the changes in the parcticipants MQ in the group, over time. A score of each movement has been made. A shorter version of BARS, BARS-8 was used. Given the time available to use the room, with BARS-8 less time for the assessment is needed. After the first BARS assessement, the patients had 20 sessions, and then, the last BARS assessment was made.

Qualitative assessment of MQ:

The study used semi-structured interviews with 3 open questions related to MQ and BBAGT. The interview was audiotaped. The interviews time range were from 30 minutes to 45 minutes. All the interviews were made the first week after the last BARS.

Open questions:

1. How do you experience with the movements?

2. How has it been the whole program in general?

3. Thinking about your daily life outside the room: Is there something useful for you coming from the therapy and how is the case.... do you use it?

To analize data the Giorgi's phenomenological method has been followed. The procedure prescribed by Giorgi is meant to embrace the total material, which due to carefull sampling consists of quite a few cases. (Malterud, K 1993)

1- To create a view of the whole. In this project: The 3 open questions related to MQ promotion

2- To identify meaningful units: listening to the tape, write down all the information and then analyze it to identify meaningful units that could fit in MQ

3- To be able to abstract the content of all the meaningful units: Place the meaningful units under their themes.

4- To gather the meaning: Looking at the original material by going backward to see if the concepts still make sense in terms of the original meaning of the interviews.

MATERIAL

The group consisted of 6 persons. One male. With an average age of 49 years. All suffering from FM and belonging to a lower socio-economic group; with a low educational level.

All the patients were referred by their family doctors to physiotherapy. They had had an average of 12 BBAT individual sessions one year before, one had 24 and 3 had no experience at all. The group had 20 sessions of BBA Group Therapy. The sessions were held in one room with enough clean and open space, light, silence and privacy; equipped with mats, chairs, and always comfortable temperature.

The twice weekly sessions had the following structure: The patients had a few minutes to meet, talk and socialize in another room with good conditions for it. After that moment, the movement session started and lasted for 75/90minutes, with the last 15 minutes for the clinical talk. The session started on the floor, taking contact with the body, and with the lying movements. Focusing on presence, starting to be``here and now,´´then continuing on to the sitting movements; keeping in mind the vertical axis and the free breathing all the time but always focusing on presence above all. It's a powerful factor, and challenging to keep it in the group. As the FM patients can feel pain or tiredness easily so it's the best way to start being in the session and be ready for the rest. Following with the standing movements: Standing balance, bouncing movement, up-down the axis, sideways, turning coordination, flexion/extension of the trunk and the arm movement. The patients could sit or lie anytime if they experienced that they needed it (but only happened two times with two different patients and for almost a minute), inviting to feel lightness and not to suffer pain, only explore it if they wanted. The individual possibilities of each patient were known from there individual therapy in the past. Enough time was used for them to repeat, explore and integrate, keeping them safe, without pushing too much and being flexible. In fact during this period of therapy they asked for a longer session (15 more minutes). The ``large jaw of the body´´ movement from Dropsy (1987) was added as there were two different aspect on the voices of the members of the group: Some more relaxed, some more rebellious during the ``AA´´sound. Most of the patients reacted with a powerful``NO´´ sound the first time they did it, so it was included after the "AA" sound movement. The session continued with relational movements, starting with the "pair movement", then the Dropsy massage, giving the patients a short moment to talk and share after each of the last two experiences. Finally: The group as a whole in the walking circle and the clinical talk. During this moment, the patients were invited to sit on the floor as Dropsy (1987) points out as something of therapeutic value for awareness.

A``contract/agreement´´was made during a previous meeting where the 6 persons interested in participating in the group were invited to come. The aims set were: Better Movement Quality, experience of health and well-being. The aims were accepted by the group. The group spontaneously, made a list with the following wishes: Balance in life, self-awareness, more vitality, gain capabilities and acceptance as a step to growth. On the contract the dates, the time and the structure of the sessions were also set. We had an open dialogue within the group, looking for understanding, agreement and commitment:``all members are involved in the process´´, ``no practicing in group outside the sessions´´, ``making a written plan for self-training´´, ``whatever was done or said during the sessions remains within the group´´. All was discussed during this meeting previous to therapy. And finally each patient signed the contract.

Ethical considerations: In the same meeting, each patient was informed verbally and in writing and also signed a consent form. The information was that the BBAGT study counted with the support of the health center, the family doctors were informed about BBAT, and all the data and results would be absolutely confidential, all names and the name of the health center and the city would be anonymous

RESULTS

The results are positive. Both: The quantitative and the qualitative.

Quantitative results

The changes in MQ scores in the 8 movements; between the first BARS and the last BARS in every patient are positive. Basic body awareness group therapy has promoted MQ in the 6 participants of the group in this study as we see on the following graphs:

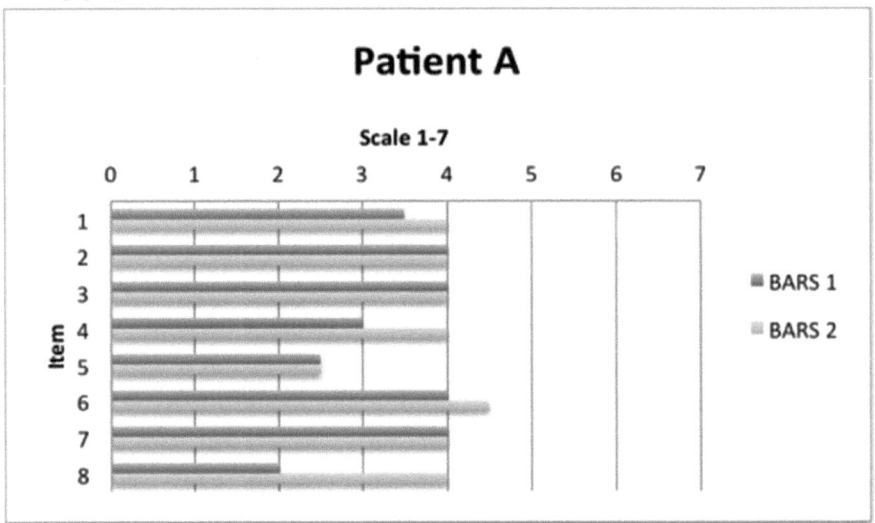

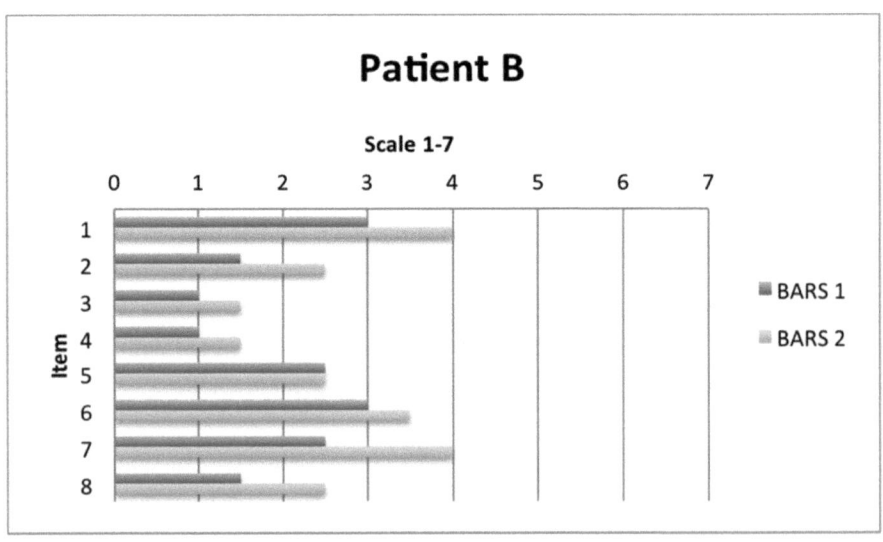

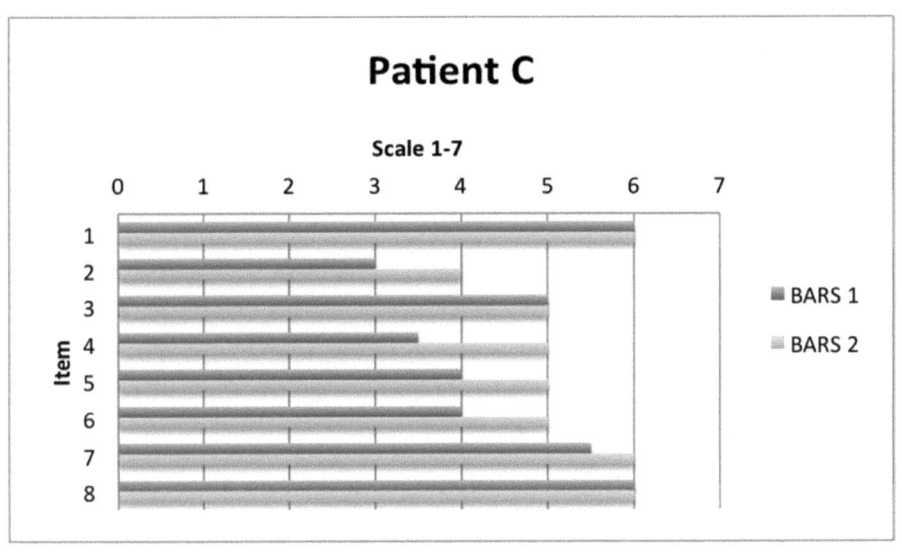

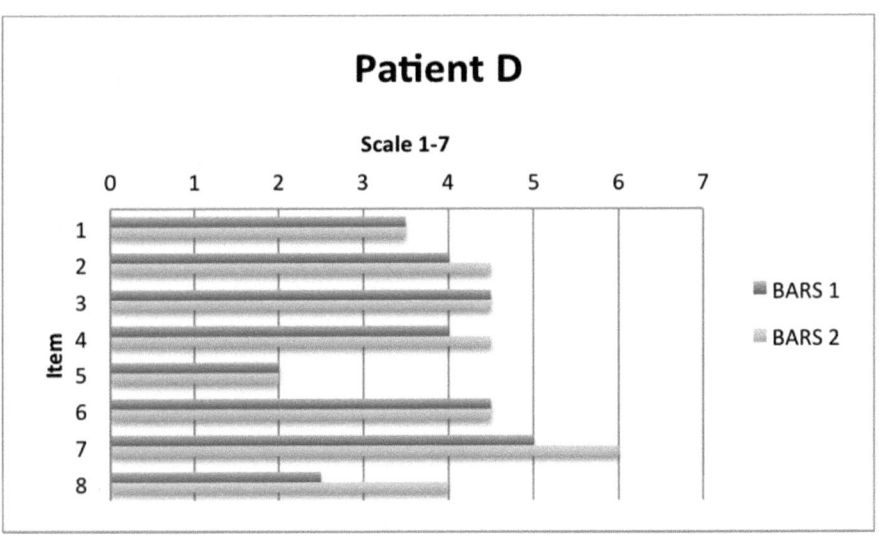

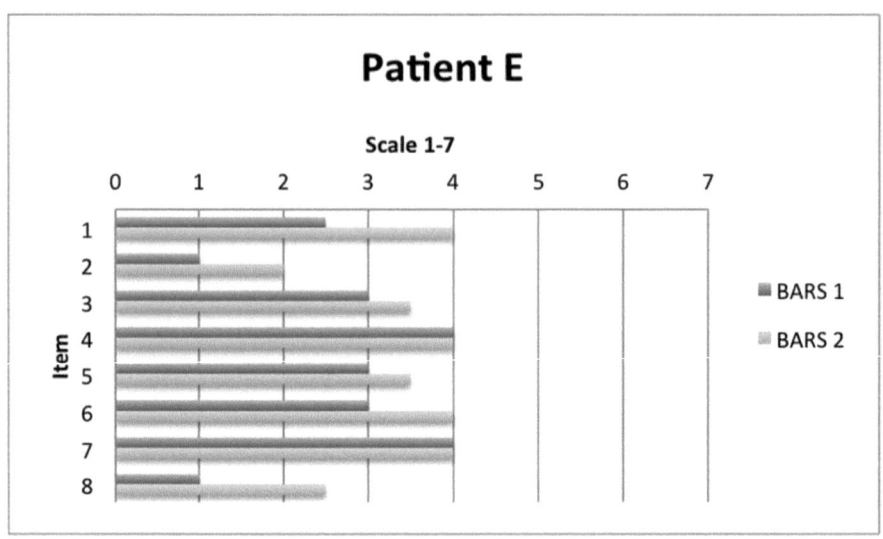

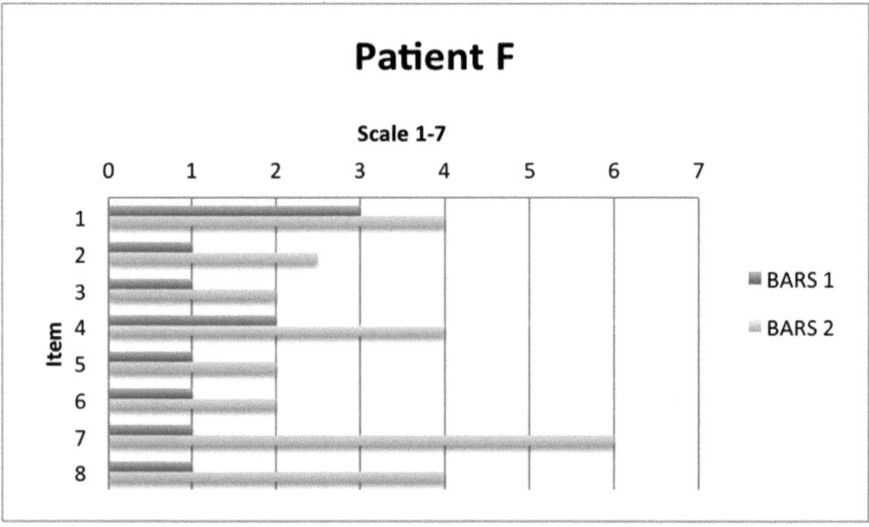

The changes if we made two average scores of the whole 8 movements in the first BARS 1 and the last BARS 2 to observe the changes in the patient with the higher level of MQ and the patient with the lowest level of MQ would show these results: Patient C (4-5), Patient F (1.5-3).

.Qualitative results: Themes

PAIN:

The patients reported less pain, more ability to control pain and even to be exploring the pain. ``I am taking no medication now´´,``I can control my pain better´´, ``I am doing experiments with the pain´´. The patients reported also less anxiety, tension and stress, but this will be seen better on the last theme.

ACCEPTANCE:

Acceptance is a concept that has been experienced by the patients in many ways: Acceptance from the therapist, acceptance to myself and FM, acceptance to personal life, acceptance from the group. ``I find acceptance and understanding by the group. Not like in the society´´,``After the whole experience I feel acceptance´´.

BODY AWARENESS:

The patients have enjoyed the therapy:``The days I have the sessions I am impatient and in a good mood. Having this sensation is important for me´´. They expressed their desire to follow with the therapy as long as possible in time. They have enjoyed the movements in general terms, experiencing the vertical axis and postural stability as something new or in some cases comfortable.``I have a better posture. I go more upright and my body feels better. People outside here sees me different and tell it to me´´. Being in the``here and now´´, has also been reported. Also harmony, being in ``the whole´´ and well-being. They have also experienced a freer breathing as one of the more powerful sources of well-being. In lying, sitting or standing, in the moments when the centre/free breathing/sound, were involved, the patients reported inner, emotional experiences:`` ``M´´ sound gives me pleasure inside me, my throat, my ears…´´,``With ``AH´´ sound, I get rid of physical weight´´, ``With ``NO´´ sound I get rid of mental weight´´. `` When lying with my hands on my centre, my body relaxes all by itself. It's not me!´´ (She refers not consciously doing it, not using her will). Also during the ``Silent movement´´: ``I feel relaxed, and I feel the sorrow from my soul. Since I was a child I had it. My mother used to tell me when she saw it in my face. But now is going away this sensation, a little…´´. Self-Awareness examples are many during the movement sessions but they will be seen on the last theme. Just one example: ``I feel that my body is walking by itself, without me doing anything´´.

THE GROUP AS A WHOLE AS AN EMBODIED LEARNING PROCESS

Many patients reported that FM isolates them from the rest of the society, feeling stigmatized. In the group they have found themselves understood, shared issues in common and felt integrated; gaining cohesion quickly. The relational movement in pairs was reported as interesting/frustrating at the beginning and finally all the patients except one, started to explore and experience in a different way; without frustration. Experiencing: ``Fun´´, ``Relaxation´´, ``A more interesting and learning experience´´. And above all: ``Something progressive´´. The Dropsy's massage was one of the favorite moments for the patients from the very first session: ``I love giving and receiving´´, `` when I receive it I feel how my body turns from concrete into rubber´´. The same happened with walking in circle when they were feeling wholeness as a group and the patients were feeling with their walking bodies moved forward by the group and in harmony. ``I feel like a rope pulling me forward´´, ``I check it. When I feel like this, I close my eyes for a moment and when I open them, my body is in harmony exactly the same´´. But the more common experience between the patients is that the group as a whole has passed through a progressive process: ``It's like a car's engine. Do you follow me?. With all the elements that are complementary to each other, and then they start to move, slowly first, then smoothly, and then little by little, faster and faster; moving the car forward´´.

WHAT HAS THE BASIC BODY AWARENESS GROUP THERAPY BROUGHT INTO MY LIFE?

In this theme: Starting from self-awareness, we see a different set of experiences. Some like: Self-control for stress, anxiety, tension, bodily self-sufficiency, self-efficiency and more capabilities, self-identity, feeling better with the familiar and social environment, more stamina, Integration of BBAT in daily life and existential issues. ``I do BBAT at home´´, ``I breathe when I need it´´, ``I use the ``here and now´´ ´´, ``I am more my ``I´´ ´´, ``I go barefoot at home´´, ``At the beginning I was skeptical. I was feeling hopeless. Now I have more physical capabilities. I am forgetting a little bit that I am chronically ill´´, ``I am more self-confident´´, ``I have no more phobia and fear to crowds, markets or lifts´´, ``I am going to be myself, I am going to develop myself as a woman..as a person´´,`` I am more myself´´, ``I am understanding my sources of stress´´, ``I am adapting the sideways movement to my repetitive movement in my job and it's energy saving´´, ``I never could do it before, but now: I stretch, sigh or yawn in public when I want; and I am feeling that I have a different attitude in life´´, ``I was very perfectionist; now I am accepting myself and my life more´´, ``Somehow I have learned to avoid tension. I tell to myself: Hillary! Are you using it for something? Stop doing it if you don't need it for anything!´´, ``what has changed is the way I move, it just flows. It's like if the movement from the room followed with me outside. BBAT is integrated in my life´´.

THE EMBODIED PRESENCE OF THE PHISIOTHERAPIST/THE GROUP LEADER

Patients perceive the therapist as somebody that provides well-being, makes the therapy something positive, promotes cohesion, and as a care-giving person. They see the therapist as an ally, helping their self-awareness. ``You have helped me to have a stronger self ´´, ``You have helped me to rediscover myself and know myself better´´. Guidance vs Correction or the Roles of ``Father/Mother´´ are perceived by the patients and they find it positive. ``I prefer our free and spontaneous therapy than gymnastics, with instructions, directions, numbers...´´ ``I like it here because I feel free but we also have discipline´´.

DISCUSSION

In this study about MQ promotion during BBAGT with 6 persons suffering from FM, the result has been found positive. In the light of the chosen theory we are going to discuss the results. Balance, free breathing and Awarenesss have improved in all the patients. The embodied presence and movement awareness of the therapist has promoted the MQ of the patients and they have reported it in many ways. Trust and acceptance and building a relationship with this 6 patients has happened from the very beginning, seing the patien´s movement resources has been a major concern of the therapist as it has been the role of ``Mother´´ and ``Father´´. In fact: At the beginning of therapy, the patients gained cohesion very quickly and the group was starting to act a bit on its own way. I realized that I was in the ``Mother role´´all the time with the group as a whole and I had to balance with the ``Father´´ role in order to gain the leadership and keep it. The patients have perceived it and found it positive. Creating the physical environment carefully, has been another important concern during therapy: The mats in ordered position, with good space, respecting the sphere of each of the patients of the session of the day, pillows on their place, and never too much or too little temperature or light. Avoiding noises and a concrete set of lights that disturbed some participants. And the chairs in an ordered position ready to be used.

Guidance vs correction has proved to work and be appreciated by the patients. Being in movement for 20 sessions for this group with past individual therapy experience has promoted changes. To be aware of the use of the therapist voice, use of the words and metaphors; tending to use less words over time has proved to be MQ promoting.

The balance between internal and external movement references of the patients has been one of the concerns during therapy, as some patients used to keep their eyes closed all the time. Sometimes I guided inviting to use all senses, but after many sessions I accepted it in some of them, keeping myself aware of their movement experience and process.

The movement awareness learning cycle has emerged as present in this study when we have in mind the focus on presence to keep the session alive and keep contact, explore and experience during the structure of the session; the patients response to the whole therapy demonstrates the existence of the other steps. It can be seen in patient's reflections in the results chapter and it has been an important MQ promoting factor.

Another perspective to discuss is relating the process of promotion of MQ with sense of coherence, and observe how SOC could have been increased during therapy and somehow is represented in the results. We will also see possible connections with some of the Yalom therapeutic factors (1985) integrated into BBAGT by Skatteboe.

We have seen in the theory chapter that there is a relationship between higher SOC and well-being between women with FM. SOC has 3 sub-dimensions. One is meaning. It refers to the extent to wich a participant feels that his or her life makes sense emotionally. (Langeland,E. 2007) Antonovsky emphasizes that this component is the most important part of SOC concept (Langeland, E. 2005). Meaning is evident in the result chapter as something experienced by the patients, and we can even connect it with the existential therapeutic factor in group therapy: When the feeling and experience is given the necessary time to integrate within the patient, it improves understanding, and gives content and meaning to his/her life. (Skatteboe 1991 in Skjaerven 2004) The general resistence resources (GRR) are crucial in the development of SOC and can be defined as any characteristic of the person, group or environment that can facilitate tension management. (Langeland, E. 2005). The GRR: Interpersonal learning, emphasizes in social support as a crucial coping resource. According to Yalom (in Skatteboe 1991 in Skjaerven 2004) interpersonal learning is the most important factor in group therapy. The group can be seen as a social microcosm. The theory of Salutogenic model insists in the function of social support to avoid losing resources and meaning over time when it talks about one of the four spheres in human life. In the GRR Cognitive and emotional, the theory stresses self-identity as a crucial coping resource.(Langeland,E. 2005)

This is not part of the result, but possibly Interpersonal learning and self-identity was observed in the group during one of the last sessions during the clinical talk. A conversation that is particularly spontaneous, unanimous and coul be interesting; that happened during the process of making this study: `` Elvis: Today it has been one of these days when you wake up with your whole body in pain. I have relaxed but the pain has been there.´^`Marilyn:``It doesn´t happen to me. I enjoy coming here but I am ok before and after. I don't have ups and downs and I do whatever I want. A little bit stiff in the morning and that's all. The doctor said I had the 18 points but maybe he was wrong and I don't have FM.´^` The group: No! No! Just there is not such a thing as FM. There are ``Fibromyalgias´´and each one``lives´´her/his FM on her/his own way´´.

Many patients reported to have integrated being in the ``here and now´´in their daily life. Presence is the hidden agent of help in all forms of therapy. ( Yalom 1985 in Skjaerven 2004) Presence and working from the principle of ``here and now´´ has been the main focus during clinical work in this study. This has possibly stimulated the group therapy therapeutic factors: Existential, interpersonal learning and group cohesion.

In the results; from the SOC perspective and concepts: It can bee seen that the patients cope better, the sub-dimension meaning is present, and coming from the GRR: Interpersonal learning, and self-identity are also included.

Now I am going to make some comments on my results. If we look at the graphs from the quantitative part of the study, the fact is that the increase in MQ has been relatively small. The patients came in general terms with a weak functional movement quality from the individual period, and the increase between the first and last BARS scores is relatively small. Certain details cannot be seen on the graphs. Patient C (appendix) has the best scores and she has the best MQ in the group. But her MQ has not been promoted so much compared with when she finished her individual treatment last year. If we see patient F, the graph is strange, she has the lowest scores and an important improvement in some movements; when the fact is that she was the patient with better MQ, from moderate to good functional MQ, the year before. She got fired from the company where she had worked for 37 years just before the first BARS in this study.

When talking with me or the other before staring, she always seemed to be in good mood. But once she entered the movement room i couldn´t help being concerned about her.

Her MQ was dysfunctional or mostly disfuntional during most of the sessions, with her eyes closed all the time and her face was like a mask with an expression of deep pain and sorrow..during all the session (except during the conversations).

It's just on the last two or three sessions and during the second BARS that her MQ started to change, her facial expression of pain disappeared, and improved quickly and this followed after the last BARS. During the interview she commented that she had realized that she had lost 37 years of her life doing something that she didn't like. And now she was going to enjoy her life and develop herself as a person. She had probably solved her ``conflict´´ in a``salutogenic´´way. I saw her MQ and her process and probably BBAGT helped, but we can't see it on her BARS score.

I have also to say that it was a bit surprising and also encouraging for me that i saw a movement quality en each of the participants of the group during all the sessions and process of group therapy with little changes in many cases but in a different situation, during the session of assasment with BARS which is individual; most of participants had a better MQ than the observed day by day on the group and somehow you realize that group work has been more fruitfull than it seemed in terms of MQ.

About the interviews, I was concerned about the fact that the patients wanted to please me as the therapist. Also, I was asking to myself about their low educational level as a difficulty for a good communication in order to get relevant information. The first concern I think didn't influenced so much. Maybe because they knew me for two years and I am also known as the physiotherapist in the neighborhood for years, so they had a ceartain feeling of ``familiarity´´ and made whatever the comments they wanted. Curiosly enough, I think that the low cultural level, in open questions, with a bit of dialogue, giving time to the patients and keeping the line of the information required a little bit; acted like an advantage. They were quite spontaneous and using their own words, images and metaphors; the interviews were quite fruitful; and a pleasant experience for both, the patients and myself.

I want to reflect about the dropouts. The initial idea was a study with more participants Only 4 patients came to 1 or 2 sessions and dropped out . This is a failure for me as therapist and group leader. They had positive reflections during the clinical talks, but they dropped out. I decided to do the project with just these 6 participants.

I believe in myself as a therapist.These concrete 6 participants in this study gained cohesion almost immediately and came regularly. They had many things in common: A past positive experience in BBAT with me. They all suffered from FM sharing many issues like stigmatization, even belonging to the same socio-economical level, the microculture of the concrete town and similar educational level. It could have reinforced the process. This subgroup well managed should have been an advantage to avoid dropouts. I ask to myself how did I fail.

At this point, I also would say that there is something purely socio-cultural to mention. With or without FM, in this part of Spain we all belong to the same culture. We have many dropouts in the physiotherapy units, specially during spring/summer. Many persons are not regular, or the socio-economic circumstances promote the dropouts.

When Eva Langeland in 2007 describes Antovsky's salutogenic theory, she points as important to be able to form a view of life (ideological, religious, or political) emphasizing in social support. And she mentions these two GRR: The Material resources; and the Macro sociocultural aspects, with an individual's culture that gives the person a place in the world and is health-promoting and where the GRR are available at different levels.

The embodied experience of pain and the suffering of millions of people persons caused by FM is very important and affects as a consequence, to our society as a whole. This has been the experienced awareness of the therapist, and the person; of the phenomenon of FM during the process that has ended in this study.

At this point: We can relate the results on this study with how another health-related science searchs to improve lives of persons suffering from FM / FMS, and how, in a very modest way; the results of promotion and increase of MQ in this group of 6 persons in this study could have been positive and coincide, to a certain extent, with part of the proposals made by this concrete researcher on her book about FM.

Our society is veri influenced by biomedicine in shaping our ideas about illness and the body.(Baker, K.K. 2005)

FMS is a socially constructed syndrome that gives meaning to a broad range of distress and suffering that characterizes the lives of many women. (Barker, K. K. 2005)

FMS represents an attempt on the part of rheumatologists to put into biomedical language women's broadly felt somatic distress; yet, in the process of translating this distress into a biomedical abstraction, the gendered basis of the abstraction was, and indeed remains, obscured.The FMS narrative gives meaning to the intergeneracional persistence of women's distress. Insofar as FMS makes sense of women's own painful lifes, it can also be applied outwardly to make sense of the similarity painful lives of women's relatives (Barker, K. K. 2005).

Unsatisfying work, including that which was low status, strenuous, and tedious, and that over which women exercised little control; characterized the occupational settings of women with FMS. With few exceptions, these women had low levels of education and work in female-dominated occupational categories.(Hallberg. Carlsson 1998 in Barker,K.K 2005)

The stories of FMS sufferers reveal complex worlds of pain-lives infused with ubiquitous and specific physical, material, and emotional hardship and suffering.(Barker, K.K 2005)

At this juncture, it might be expected the presentation of the standard social science and feminist critique of biomedicine and demand that it be more attentive to the social forces that shape women´s health. (Baker, K.K. 2005)

In a culture that promotes the dual ideologies of individualism and meritocracy, FMS functions as one of the few available explanations for the everyday and dramatic suffering that marks many women´s lives, including that which persist across generations of women. In a culture that cannot see how personal troubles might be public issues.(Barker, K.K 2005)

In short, by medicalizing such a broad assortment of human suffering, FMS runs the risk to either anestehetizing or depoliticizing women's everyday lifes. (Barker,K.K. 2005)

We require an awareness of the cultural dominance of biomedicine, both as a set of beliefs and as an institution. In our society, biomedical principles, metaphors and ideals provide the dominant framework through which embodied reality is experienced and given meaning. We assume that biomedicine has the capacity to alter the course of nature and that the ``normal´´ state of nature is the absence of suffering. (Barker,K.K. 2005)

According with many researchers, FM seems nonexistent in indigenous cultures such as those in Africa or in China.

Cultural aspects matter in BBAT/MQ. It´s just a reflection while we follow Barker's theories (mostly based and developed from studies and research made in developed countries).

In the case of FMS, the underrepresentation of black women is found not only in the clinical context but also in community prevalence studies studies that are not biased by racial differences in acces to health care .(Barker, K.K. 2005) Part of the cultural disposition of many black women may be a tendency toward the routinization and normalization of pain (broadly defined). (Barker, K.K. 2005)

As a result of the persistence of gender, race, and class inequality, contemporary black women remain unlikely to experience their distress and comprised well-being as a "problem that has no name". More than 10 years ago, the National Black Women´s Health Project and The Black Women´s Health Book (White 1990) brought this perspective to the fore.(Barker,K.K. 2005)

There is an explanation for the majority of white, working and lower middle-class women among those with FMS. Compared with more affluent white women, they share the dominant cultural expectation of a life free from pain, but they lack the resources with which to realize that norm. Yet compared with black and other minority women, they also lack a cultural understanding that normalizes the resulting suffering and gives it a social meaning. Within their cultural world, suffering is unexpected and unexplainable. FMS, therefore, is associated with genuine suffering that is rooted in the material condition of women's lives, but is also dependent on a disposition in which women see themselves as entitled to painless and biomedicine as a route to that entitlement (Barker, K K 2005)

We must become less dependent on biomedicine for making sense of our lives and our suffering. We need to be more sociological, multidimensional, and intellectually creative ourselves. We need to politicize the ways that social and economic forces impact the well-being of those who are relatively disempowered, knowing full well that those forces and their effects cannot be captured biomedically. We need to produce a public narrative that makes sense of pain and distress as grounded in the everyday fabric of women's (and men's) lives and that directs our energies toward the search for solutions beyond the realm of biomedicine (Barker, K.K. 2005).

Biomedicine is very needed, and like any other discipline involved in health, is related to the power as is normal in society. Analyzing this question or the particular vision of Kristin K. Barker is not part of this discussion.

But Yalom sees the group as a social microcosm, and the increase and promotion of MQ has showed in this 6 persons microcosm: A better relationship to others and increased self- awareness and self-reflection in many areas of life. And I would insist: Meaning and an increased SOC could be`` observed´´ thru the reading of the pages of this study.

BBAT is salutogenic and has humanistic principles. BBAT is multidimensional. I have even seen creativity in movement in one of my patients. With BBAGT it has been made a very modest contribution to the well-being of 6 persons suffering from FM, to society, and maybe, to part of what social science could propose to reduce the suffering of persons with FM. Just in this study with this very little group of women (and a man). Even if we don't know for how long.

Dropsy described the 3-fold contact problem as a lack of awareness of the physical body and internal life, of the physical environment, and of the relationship to other people. (Skjaerven, L. H. et al 2010)

Strengthening the self-awareness increases the opportunities to self-experience and self-reflection in all areas of life. (Dropsy 1988; Mattsson 1998 in Skjaerven et al 2008).

Positive experiences of the body were intertwined with a new relationship to self and objects in the world. Interactions between the co-participants promoted the process of creating new patterns of thinking and acting in the social world .(Mannerkorpi, K. Gard, G. 2003)

Eliminating risk factors are less impotant in sustaining health than having acces to factors of health. (Mattsson,M. et al 2000)

CONCLUSION

The Movement quality has been promoted and increased during Basic Body Awareness Group Therapy in this study with a group of 6 persons suffering from Fibromyalgia.

The results are posititive and indicate that MQ promotion and increase in BBAGT can improve health-related quality of life in this group of persons suffering from fibromyalgia.

Quite possibly the fact that all the 6 participants on the group therapy had a past positive experience with individual Basic Body Awareness Therapy, has facilitated, the promotion of MQ during group therapy, and the results of this study.

This project has ment for me an important growth as a professional and as a person and the opportunity to be, relate, and have a bodily contact with persons suffering from fibromyalgia, learning a lot about human suffering. This makes me feel more prepared as a physiotherapist for any patient.

In a larger project: I woul like to be part of a multidisciplinary study. In the same context: Primary care, health centre, public health and in the same social and cultural environment. I am saying Spain. This way, the experience I have from this study, could be useful.

And ideally: Being part of a team counting with the Spanish family doctor and psychoanalist Santiago Castellanos, who is being 12 years doing research in FM in the exact same context.

Another project that catches my interest and imagination and I found challenging, would be with a multidisciplinary study with similar caractheristics, quantitative and qualitative but this time with men as most of the persons that suffer this concrete health´s problem.

Unavoidably during all my research i have found a "family" of functional somatic syndromes or defined with different, words depending on the researcher.

Obviously I am talking about the Gulf War Illness.

As a researcher, thinking in grouptherapy, empathy is a must and in the phenomeologycal cualitative research aspect, the researcher is part of the phenomenon studied and empathy once again I think, is the key to "be in" it.

I would spend a period of time "on the field", maybe serving in a military healthcare unit, and after, I would start the study in the home land of these men.

But this is another story....

REFFERENCES

Antonovsky A.(1987) Unraveling the mystery of health. How people manage stress and stay well. Jossey-Bass.1987

Van Den Berg (2011) Science and Research Methodology and Methods. Class during Block 1, BBAM, HiB. Bergen. Norway.

 Langeland, E et al (2007) Promoting coping: Salutogenesis among people with mental health problems. Included in: Sense of Coherence and Life in People suffering from Mental Health Problems. An intervention study in talk-therapy with focus in salutogenesis. Dissertation for degree doctor rerum politicarum.University of Bergen.Norway

Skjaerven LH, Gard G, Kristoffersen K (2008) An Eye for Movement Quality : A Phenomenological Study of Movement Quality reflecting a Group of Physiotherapist´s Understanding of the Phenomenon. Physiotherapy Theory and Practice, 24(1): 13-27. INFORMA Healthcare.

 Skjaerven, LH, Kristoffersen K, Gard G (2010) How can Movement Quality be Promoted in Clinical Practice? A Phenomenological Study of Physical Therapy Experts. American Physical Therapy Association.

 Van der Kolk, BA, Mc Farlane AC, Weisaeth, L (1996) Traumatic Stress. The effects of Overwhelming Experiences on Mind, Body and Society. Chap 1 and 2

 Mannerkorpy K, Gard G (2003) Physiotherapy Group Treatment for patients with Fibromyalgia-an Embodied learning process. Disability and Rehabilitation, Vol. 25, NO. 24.

 Gard G (2005) Body Awareness Therapy for Patients With Fibromyalgia and Chronic Pain. Disability and Rehabilitation, 27(129: 725-728. Taylor & Francis.

 Hammel KW (2004) Using Qualitative Evidence as a Basis for Evidence-Based Practice. In Qualitative Research in Evidence-Based Rehabitlitation (ed K. W. Hammel, Carpenter, C)

 Malterud K (1993) Shared Understanding of the Qualitative Research Process. Guidelines for the Medical Researcher. Family Practice, 10, No.2, 201-206

 Skjaerven, LH (2002) Basic Body Awareness Therapy. Exercises, verbal guidance, observation and assessment of Quality of Movement. A first Introduction.

 Skatteboe, UB (2005) Basic Body Awareness Therapy and Movement Harmony. Development of BARS-MH. Oslo University College.

 Skjaerven LH (2004) Being in dialogue. Basic Body Awareness in Group Therapy. Level III.

Yalom I D (1995) The Theory and Practice of Group Psychotherapy (3rd ed) New York: Basic Books. Chap. 1

Skjaerven, LH (2003) Basic Body Awareness Therapy. A guide to understanding,therapy and growth. Level II

Mattsson M, Wilkman M, Dahlgren L, Mattsson B (2000) Physiotherapy as Empowerment-Treating Women with Chronic Pelvic Pain. Advances in Physiotherapy; 2: 125-143

Barker K.K. (2005) The Fibromyalgia Story. Medical Authority and Women's worlds of pain. Temple University Press. Philadelphia. Introduction, chap.1, 2, 3, 4, 5, 7, 8, conclusion

Castellanos S. (2012) El Dolor y los Lenguajes del Cuerpo. Grama Ediciones. Buenos Aires. Introduction, chap 1, chap 2, chap 4,chap 5.

Cunnningham, M.M. (2006) Individuals'descriptions of Living with Fibromyalgia. Clinical Nursing Research. Vol 15, Number 4

Hasset, A.L., Clauw,D.J. (2011) Does Psychological Stress cause Chronic Pain?. Psychiatric Clinics of North America, 34, 579-594. Elsevier Inc.

Bergman, S. (2005) Psychosocial aspects of Chronic Widespread Pain and Fibromyalgia. Disability and Rehabilitation. Taylor & Francis Group Ltd.

Soderverg, S. Lundman, B. Norberg,A. (1997) Living with Fibromyalgia: Sense of Coherence, Perception of Well-Being, and Stress in Daily life. Research in Nursing & Health, 20, 495-503. John Wiley & Sons, Inc.

Przekop, P. et al (2010) Correlates of Perceived Pain-Related Restrictions among Women with Fibromyalgia. Pain Medicine 11, 1698-1706. Willey Periodicals Inc.

Smith, B.W. et al (2009) Traumatic Events, Perceived Stress and Health in Women with Fibromyalgia and Healthy Controls. Stress and Health.John. Wiley & Sons, Ltd.

Mannerkorpi, K. Gard,G. (2003) Physiotherapy Group Treatment for Patients with Fibromyalgia-an Embodied Learning Process. Disability and Rehabilitation. Vol. 25,no 24, 1372-1380. Taylor & Francis Ltd.

National Fibromyalgia Partnership, Inc.(2005). FM Monograph. Fibromyalgia: Symptoms, Diagnosis, Treatment & Research.www.fmpartnership.org

Cohen, H. et al (2002) Prevalence of Post-Traumatic Stress Disorder in Fibromyalgia Patients: Overlapping Syndromes or Post-Traumatic Fibromyalgia Syndrome? Seminars in Arthritis and Rheumatism, vol 32, 38-50. Elsevier Science.

Undeland, M. Malterud(2007) The Fibromyalgia Diagnosis-Hardly Helpful for the Patients? Scandinavian Journal of Primary Health Care. Taylor&Francis.

Raheim, M. Haland, W. (2006) Lived Experience of Chronic Pain and Fibromyalgia: Women's Stories From Daily Life. Qualitative Health Research. Stage Publications

Zavestoski, S. et al (2004) Patient Activism and the Struggle for Diagnosis: Gulf War Illnesses and other Medically Unexplained Physical Symptoms in the US. Social Science & Medicine 58, 161-175. Elsevier Science Ltd.

Morea, J.M. Friend, R. Bennett, R.M. (2008) Conceptualizing and Measuring Illness Self-Concept: A Comparison in Predicting Fibromyalgia Adjustment. Research in Nursing & Health 31, 563-575. Wiley Periodicals, Inc.

Murray Jr. T.L. et al (2007) Stress and Family Relationship Functioning as Indicators of the Severity of Fibromyalgia Symptoms: A Regression Analysis. Stress and Health 23, 3-8. John Wiley & Sons, Ltd.

Amanda Lundvik Gyllensten. (2001) Basic Body Awareness Therapy. In Department of Physical Therapy. Lund: Lund University. Sweden

Skjaerven LH, Gard, G, Kristoffersen, k. (2008). An Eye for Movement Quality : A Phenomenological Study of Movement Quality reflecting a Group of Physiotherapist´s Understanding of the Phenomenon. Physiotherapy Theory and Practice

Martinsen, k. (2006). Care and Vulnerability. Akribe. Chap 4-(Evidence in health care)

Marcus, D. A. Deodhar, A. (2011). Fibromyalgia. A Practical Clinical Guide. Springer Science+Business Media.

Ventedgot, S. Gringols, M. Merrick, J. (2005). Clinical Holistic Medicine: Whiplash, Fibromyalgia, and Chronic Fatigue. The Scientific World Journal.

Mas, A. J. Carmona, L. Valverde, M. Ribas, B. and EPISER Study Group. (2008) Prevalence and Impact of Fibromyalgia on Function and Quality of life. Life in Individuals from a Nationwide Study in Spain. Clinical and Experimental Rheumatology.

Kool, M. B. Geenen, R. (2011). Loneliness in Patients with Rheumatic Diseases: The Significance of Invalidation and Lack of Social Support. The Journal of Psychology: Interdisciplinary and Applied.

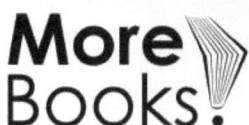
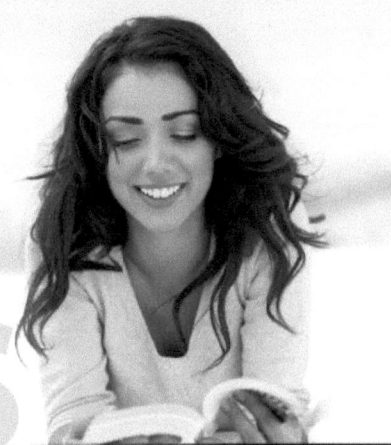

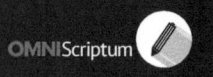

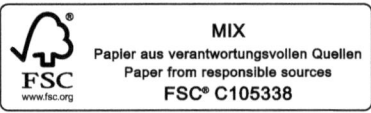
Printed by Books on Demand GmbH, Norderstedt / Germany